AF884588

THE MEDICINE-FREE,

ILLNESS-FREE SERIES

INTEGRATIVE THERAPIES FOR EVERYDAY HEALTH

Science-Informed and User-Trusted Solutions

Forest Yin, DAOM, L.Ac.

Ashi Healing Publishing

Copyright © 2025 by Dr. Forest Yin

All rights reserved.

No part of this book may be reproduced, stored, or transmitted in any form or by any means—electronic, mechanical, photocopying, recording, or otherwise—without prior written permission from the publisher, except for brief quotes used in reviews.

First Edition: May 2025

Published by Ashi Healing

www.AshiHealing.com

Paperback ISBN: 978-1-967735-18-1

eBook ISBN: 978-1-967735-19-8

Printed in the United States of America

Medical Disclaimer:

This book is for informational purposes only and is not intended as medical advice. The author and publisher assume no responsibility for how the information is used. Readers should consult a healthcare professional before making any health-related decisions.

Foreword

Nature is the origin of life, the origin of healing, and remains a guiding force in human well-being. Long before modern science developed medicine in laboratories, nature provided everything the human body needed to survive, and to sustain life. The food we eat, the herbs we gather, the minerals beneath our feet, and the sun above us are all part of an intelligent and interconnected system that has long nourished and supported the human body.

This truth has been known across cultures for thousands of years, and it is echoed in sacred texts. In the Book of Genesis, the Garden of Eden was described as a paradise where "every tree that is pleasant to the sight and good for food" was made available to humankind (Genesis 2:9). Some scholars believe this refers not only to nourishment, but also to the ability to contribute to human well-being. It becomes even more clear in Ezekiel 47:12: "The fruit thereof shall be for meat, and the leaf thereof for medicine."

Somewhere along the way, modern culture drifted from this wisdom. Many now believe that healing must come through synthetic drugs, surgeries, or man-made interventions, forgetting that the foundation of human health has always been rooted in nature. But what if well-being isn't only about medical breakthroughs, but also about reconnecting with what has always been available to us?

What if the body doesn't need to be forced to function differently, but simply supported, nourished, balanced, and reminded of what it already knows? What if illness is not the enemy, but a signal that we've fallen out of balance, and out of sync with nature?

This is not to dismiss the value of conventional medicine. We are deeply grateful for its life-saving capabilities in emergencies and acute care. But when it comes to supporting long-term vitality and encouraging balance, it may be time to return to the source.

In addition to thousands of years of lived wisdom, modern science is now exploring the potential of many natural approaches. What was once viewed as "alternative" is now increasingly recognized as part of a broader wellness conversation.

This book, and the entire *Medicine-Free, Illness-Free Series*, is rooted in this truth:

Nature not only gave us life. Many believe it holds the power to support our well-being. And many of these natural approaches are now being studied and better understood through science.

Healing is not something we must force or fear. It is something we can encourage, by gently supporting the body, naturally.

Dr. Forest Yin, DAOM, L.Ac.

Author, *The Medicine-Free, Illness-Free Series*

Founder, Ashi Healing and Acupuncture Inc.

Important Disclaimer

The supplements, therapies, and natural approaches discussed in *The Medicine-Free, Illness-Free Series* are intended to support general wellness and the body's natural balance. They are not intended to diagnose, treat, cure, or prevent any disease and have not been evaluated by the U.S. Food and Drug Administration (FDA).

These books are provided for educational purposes only and are not a substitute for professional medical advice, diagnosis, or treatment. Always consult your physician or a licensed healthcare provider before starting any new supplement, therapy, or wellness routine, especially if you are pregnant, nursing, have a medical condition, or are taking medications.

The content in this series is informed by two sources: summaries of available scientific research, presented as "Science-Informed Solution Benefits", and aggregated user feedback, presented as "Customer-Reported Solution Benefits". These are intended to inform and inspire, but they reflect general patterns, not guarantees. Individual results will vary.

The phrase *"Medicine-Free, Illness-Free"* reflects a natural wellness philosophy and is not a medical claim or promise of outcome.

By reading this book, you agree to take full responsibility for your personal health choices and to seek guidance from qualified health professionals when needed.

Contents

Preface

Do you feel like you've tried everything—medications, conventional treatments, even supplements—yet still struggle with fatigue, discomfort, brain fog, or other daily wellness concerns?

If so, you're not alone.

Many people today are turning to nature-based solutions, not as replacements for essential medical care, but as gentle, sustainable ways to support their overall well-being.

The rise in chronic health challenges reflects this shift. According to the CDC, over 60% of U.S. adults live with at least one chronic health condition, and more than 40% manage two or more. More than 40% of school-aged children in the United States are reported to have at least one ongoing wellness concern, rising sharply in recent years.

At the same time, modern habits, nutrient-depleted diets, environmental stressors, and sedentary routines, have created a disconnect between how we live and what the body truly needs to stay resilient. For many, conventional solutions haven't fully addressed these patterns, leaving people still searching for support that feels both effective and sustainable.

That's what *The Medicine-Free, Illness-Free Series* is here to explore.

This series introduces practical, natural options that may help support energy, digestion, sleep, focus, mood, and more, without requiring major lifestyle changes or complicated routines.

It doesn't reject conventional medicine. It expands your toolkit. While modern treatments often focus on managing symptoms in the short term, natural health practices are designed to work more gradually, supporting the body's natural rhythms over time. Many people are rediscovering how ancient practices and modern science can work together, not in opposition, to create a more balanced, resilient life.

The Medicine-Free, Illness-Free Series is built on two foundational pillars:

Science-Informed Solution Benefits: exploring what modern research says about the potential benefits associated with each supplement or therapy

Customer-Reported Solution Benefits: drawn from thousands of real-world user feedback to highlight what people most often experience in practice, including common benefit themes, typical use case patterns, and key user insights.

By combining scientific research with traditional use and real-world user feedback, each volume empowers you to make informed decisions, grounded in both evidence and everyday reality.

Each book in the series focuses on one category of natural therapies. Whether you're exploring Herbal Therapy, Mushroom Therapy, Amino Acid support, Animal Organ Supplements, Grounding, the HOPED Protocol, or detoxification, the goal is the same: to offer trusted solutions that fit easily into your life, simply, naturally, and sustainably.

You don't need to overhaul your lifestyle or commit to an elaborate health plan. You can begin right where you are. Even one small step, a single herb, nutrient, or daily practice, can help you create a rhythm of care that supports your body more naturally over time.

Preface

While no approach guarantees results, many people have found these natural strategies helpful in supporting comfort, energy, focus, and overall vitality. This series was created to help you explore those tools with clarity and confidence, without pressure or complexity.

This volume focuses on Integrative Therapies for Everyday Health, offering practical insight into science-informed and user-trusted solutions for common wellness goals. You'll explore a wide range of approaches through both research and real-world perspectives, so you can decide what feels right for your journey.

Thank you for beginning this exploration.

Let's move forward, one natural step at a time.

The Medicine-Free, Illness-Free Series

The Medicine-Free, Illness-Free Series is your go-to resource for practical, research-informed natural strategies that are easy to apply. Each volume focuses on a single modality or system—herbs, mushrooms, organ supplements, amino acids, grounding, detox, and more—offering clear guidance to help you choose what works best for you.

Together, the 10 books provide a comprehensive yet flexible wellness framework that supports both daily health maintenance and targeted support. Here's a brief overview of what you'll find in each book:

The Medicine-Free, Illness-Free Series: Why Natural Health Is the Future

Explore why millions of people are turning to nature-aligned strategies to support their wellness. This foundational volume introduces the core science and philosophy behind natural approaches to health, and how they may support your sense of balance, vitality, and overall well-being.

The Medicine-Free, Illness-Free Series: Herbal Therapy

Learn how the world's most time-tested plants may support digestion, energy, relaxation, immune strength, and more. Discover practical ways to include them in your routine and how to choose herbs that match your personal needs and constitution.

The Medicine-Free, Illness-Free Series: Mushroom Therapy

Discover the unique compounds found in medicinal mushrooms that may support immunity, cognitive function, and stress resilience. This book explains how to use mushrooms such as Reishi, Lion's Mane, and Cordyceps in a daily supplement.

The Medicine-Free, Illness-Free Series: Animal Organ Therapy

Explore how nutrient-dense organ supplements, like liver, heart, and kidney, may provide highly bioavailable vitamins, minerals, and peptides. Learn how these traditional foods may support foundational wellness in areas like energy, endurance, and metabolic balance.

The Medicine-Free, Illness-Free Series: Amino Acid Therapy

Uncover the role of amino acids, the building blocks of life, in supporting mood, focus, muscle strength, and nervous system health. This volume shows how targeted amino acid support may help restore clarity, resilience, and emotional well-being.

The Medicine-Free, Illness-Free Series: HOPED Protocol

Learn the five foundational nutrient categories—High Fiber, Omega-3s & Antioxidants, Probiotics, Enzymes, and Vitamin D—and how to implement them as a core wellness strategy. HOPED is simple, actionable, and designed for everyday consistency.

The Medicine-Free, Illness-Free Series: Detoxification Therapy

Discover a gentle, nature-based approach to support your body's natural detoxification processes, promote balance, and encourage overall vitality using simple, practical techniques.

The Medicine-Free, Illness-Free Series: Grounding Therapy

Explore the science and practice of grounding (earthing), the natural process of reconnecting with the Earth's electrical field. Learn how this subtle practice may help support nervous system regulation, sleep quality, and emotional balance.

The Medicine-Free, Illness-Free Series: Diet, Lifestyle and Emotional Well-being

While drastic changes are not required, this volume introduces simple habits that promote long-term balance, covering food, movement, sleep, and emotional self-regulation in a way that aligns with the rest of your natural health plan.

The Medicine-Free, Illness-Free Series: Integrative Therapies for Everyday Health

This final volume brings together insights from the entire series, offering user-reported tools to help support everyday wellness goals, such as energy, digestion, sleep, immunity, and emotional resilience. It serves as a cross-reference for applying the therapies in complementary ways, helping you navigate your health journey with clarity and confidence.

Meet Dr. Forest Yin, DAOM, L.Ac.

Professionally known as Forest Yin, my official name is Jie Yin, while also known as 尹明杰 in the Chinese speaking communities.

For most of my professional life, I was known as a high-tech executive, problem-solver, and innovator in information security and technologies. In leadership roles at Oracle, Schwab, and Wells Fargo, I developed and managed advanced security solutions, ensuring stability, efficiency, and high performance in a fast-paced, high-stakes environment.

But after work, I was deeply immersed in another world, the science of natural health.

My journey into Traditional Chinese Medicine (TCM) began in college, when I first studied the *Huang Di Nei Jing (Yellow Emperor's Classic of Internal Medicine)* alongside my Physics degree. While excelling in my tech career, I continued to research, experiment, and apply natural healing principles, seeking ways to optimize health, energy, and resilience, not just for myself, but for those around me.

Recognizing the profound impact of natural medicine on long-term health and performance, I pursued formal training, becoming a Licensed Acupuncturist (L.Ac.) in 2018 and earning my Doctorate in Acupuncture and Oriental Medicine (DAOM) in 2019. Since then, I have supported individuals around the world in improving their vitality, resilience, and sense of well-being through natural methods. This led me to found Ashi Healing and Acupuncture Inc. and become a Professor and Doctoral Advisor at the University of East-West Medicine, where I mentor future practitioners in the art of TCM.

Applying Systems Thinking to Health & Healing

In high-tech, solving problems requires understanding systems, identifying vulnerabilities, and optimizing performance. I apply the same mindset to health. Instead of treating symptoms, I look at the root cause, like debugging a system. Instead of temporary fixes, I focus on long-term balance and resilience, like designing sustainable architecture. Instead of pharmaceutical dependency, I seek efficient, natural approaches that support function and balance gently, without the common side effects associated with conventional options, like optimizing system performance.

While many of my colleagues in the tech and finance industries thrived in their careers, I also saw the toll of chronic stress, burnout, autoimmune conditions, and lifestyle-related illnesses. Like many professionals, they pushed their limits, until their bodies pushed back. This is where natural approaches can make a difference.

A Philosophy Rooted in Balance & Natural Healing

At Ashi Healing, my approach complements conventional care by focusing on identifying underlying imbalances and supporting the body's natural self-regulation through Traditional Chinese Medicine and holistic strategies.

The name "Ashi (阿是)" comes from a fundamental concept in Chinese medicine, that moment of realization when healing feels real. In Chinese, "Ashi" means "Ahh, Yes!", the instant when your body recognizes exactly what it needs. This guiding philosophy shapes everything I do, from acupuncture to natural health solutions.

Through the precise use of Chinese Herbal Medicine and modern whole-food-based natural supplements like herbs and mushrooms, I have helped individuals support their energy and balance naturally, using simple, sustainable tools that complement or reduce the need for pharmaceutical interventions when appropriate.

My mission is simple: to help people pursue wellness and resilience, naturally and sustainably.

Integrating Ancient Wisdom with Modern Innovation

Chinese Herbal Medicine has been refined for thousands of years. But today, we can take it further, combining ancient wisdom with modern research and a strategic, data-driven approach to health optimization.

At Ashi Healing, I personalize each protocol based on the individual's needs, whether it's boosting energy, reducing stress, improving cognitive function, or addressing chronic health concerns. Many of the people I work with are busy professionals seeking practical, time-efficient strategies to support their health without disrupting their demanding schedules.

Looking for More Information and Support

To learn more about my personalized approach to Chinese Herbal Therapy and whole-food-based supplements, visit AshiHealing.com. You'll find additional resources and simple ways to take the next step in your healing journey, whenever you're ready.

And remember, this book is just one part of *The Medicine-Free, Illness-Free Series*. Each volume explores a different pillar of natural healing, from herbs and mushrooms to amino acids, detoxification, and grounding, offering you a complete path to support your balance and well-being through nature-based strategies.

A Science-Backed, Real-World Tested Method

In *The Medicine-Free, Illness-Free Series*, we introduce a unique, structured method for exploring natural supplements, one that blends scientific insight with real-world observations. Rather than relying solely on clinical studies or anecdotal reports, we combine both perspectives to give you a well-rounded, user-friendly understanding of each natural solution.

This balanced approach helps answer the most important questions: What does science suggest about this supplement's potential? What are people actually experiencing when they use it? Which health goals do people turn to it for most often?

Our method reflects a commitment to transparency, education, and practicality, so you can explore these natural options with clarity and confidence.

Our Four-Part Analysis Method

1. Science-Informed Solution Benefits

We begin by reviewing peer-reviewed studies, traditional usage patterns, and emerging scientific literature to understand the possible mechanisms and effects of each supplement. This provides a foundation of what is known, hypothesized, or being actively researched, offering a science-informed perspective to guide your exploration.

2. Customer-Reported Solution Benefits

We analyze large sets of customer reviews from publicly available platforms to understand how these supplements are being used in daily life. This includes what benefits people say they notice most often and how they describe their experiences.

Our focus is on patterns of what users commonly report, rather than isolated stories. This real-world layer helps connect the theory to practical, everyday outcomes.

3. Use Case Patterns & Feedback Insights

Within the customer-reported section, we highlight:

Use Case Patterns Observed – What kinds of goals or wellness concerns people most commonly use each supplement for.

Feedback Insights – How users describe the impact in their own words, including sentiment, language tone, and satisfaction cues.

Most Reported Benefits – A percentage-based summary showing which benefits are mentioned most often in reviews.

This structured summary lets you see what real people are using the supplement for, and how frequently those benefits are reported.

4. No Brand Promotion—Just Trusted Guidance

This series does not promote specific products or brands. Instead, we offer education and a decision-making framework. For those looking for high-quality sources, recommended supplement types and vetted options are available at AshiHealing.com.

Why This Method Matters

In today's crowded supplement market, it can be hard to separate hype from helpful information. That's why we created this approach, to empower you with insights drawn from scientific research, real-world usage patterns and satisfaction trends, and clear summaries that help you compare options and set expectations

You won't find exaggerated claims or one-size-fits-all solutions here. Instead, you'll find a practical, transparent method that reflects how real people are exploring natural wellness, with science as a guide and personal experience as a reference.

Whether you're considering herbs, mushrooms, amino acids, or other supplements, this method gives you a safe and structured way to learn how others are using these tools, and how they might fit into your own wellness journey.

A Personal Commitment from Dr. Forest Yin

Every approach, strategy, and supplement featured in *The Medicine-Free, Illness-Free Series* has been personally explored. Before sharing any recommendations with clients or readers, I take the time to experience it myself, observing how it affects energy, mood, sleep, digestion, and focus.

This hands-on approach allows me to understand each therapy not just through science, or just through other people's experiences. It adds a personal layer of insight to the research and user-reported feedback that shape this series.

My goal is simple: to help you find natural, sustainable solutions that feel doable, helpful, and aligned with how lasting wellness begins, by reconnecting with your body's own rhythms and innate intelligence.

How to Use This Book

This book is your practical, easy-to-navigate guide to exploring trusted natural solutions for everyday health goals. It draws from both scientific insight and the experiences of thousands of real-world users, helping you discover which natural therapies people turn to most often, what they use them for, and why they're widely trusted.

Start with What You Need

Begin by identifying your wellness goal or area of concern. The Table of Contents is organized by body systems, such as immune, digestive, or cognitive health, with commonly mentioned issues and goals listed under each. Whether you're looking to feel more energized, sleep more soundly, improve focus, or support digestion, you'll be able to quickly find the relevant section.

Explore Trusted Solutions from Across the Series

For each health goal, you'll find natural solutions featured in *The Medicine-Free, Illness-Free Series*, carefully selected based on two criteria: scientific rationale and consistently positive user feedback.

These include therapies from the full series:

Herbal Therapy – Widely used botanicals studied for their supportive potential

Mushroom Therapy – Functional mushrooms noted for immune and vitality support

Animal Organ Therapy – Nutrient-rich supplements inspired by ancestral nutrition

Amino Acid Therapy – Key building blocks for metabolism, strength, and mood

HOPED Protocol – Foundational nutrients like Omega-3s, enzymes, and Vitamin D

Detoxification Therapy – Natural ingredients used to support internal cleansing

Grounding Therapy – Gentle reconnection with Earth's natural energy

Only the most widely used and positively reviewed solutions are featured. In most cases, each solution holds an average satisfaction rating of 4.5 stars or higher, based on public reviews. While this isn't a guarantee of effectiveness, it signals that many people find them helpful and easy to integrate into their wellness routines.

What Makes This Approach Unique

Rather than focusing solely on clinical trial data, this book highlights insights from tens of thousands of users who have shared their real-world experiences. These insights are organized into a framework called **Customer-Reported Benefits**, based on what people most frequently mention in 4- and 5-star reviews.

We calculate something called a **Benefit Share (%)**, the percentage of positive reviews that mention a specific benefit. For example, if 67% of users mention immune support when reviewing Astragalus, that's a strong signal that it's a common experience. Similarly, Turkey Tail may show a 30% share for immune resilience during seasonal transitions.

These percentages help you quickly understand:

What benefits people report most often

Which wellness goals a supplement is most commonly used for

How consistent the experiences tend to be across a wide range of users

This user-driven perspective empowers you to set realistic expectations and make more informed choices, especially if you're exploring natural health solutions for the first time.

Science-Informed, Not Just Anecdotal

Each entry is also supported by scientific context that helps explain why these solutions may be beneficial. For example, Astragalus is known for its immunomodulatory properties in laboratory studies, while compounds in Turkey Tail, such as PSK, have been studied for their ability to support immune function.

By combining science-informed reasoning with high-volume user insights, you get a well-rounded picture of each therapy's potential, grounded in both research and reality.

Why the Full Series Matters

While this book offers a quick-reference overview, the real depth of understanding comes from reading each therapy book in *The Medicine-Free, Illness-Free Series.* Each one provides a more complete picture, explaining the science behind how the solutions work, how people actually describe their experiences, and how you can use them safely and effectively. If you want to make informed, confident decisions and truly understand what these natural solutions can offer, taking the time to explore the full series will be one of the most valuable steps you can take for your health.

Your Health, Your Choice

This book was created to support and simplify your wellness journey, without requiring extreme routines or guesswork. Whether you're seeking to feel more energized, improve digestion, enhance focus, or support your immune system, this guide offers tools that are both grounded in science and trusted by everyday users.

Let's explore the most trusted, science-informed natural therapies that may support your everyday health goals, safely, naturally, and with clarity.

Immune System Support

Your immune system is responsible for protecting your body from infections, harmful pathogens, and abnormal cells that may disrupt healthy function. A strong and well-regulated immune response is essential for maintaining health, supporting recovery from illness, and promoting long-term resilience.

However, many factors in modern life such as chronic stress, poor nutrition, environmental toxins, and insufficient quality sleep can negatively impact immune function. When the immune system is compromised, individuals may experience more frequent illnesses, slower recovery, increased inflammation, or reduced overall vitality.

Fortunately, natural therapies may help enhance and regulate immune function, offering sustained support for immune balance and daily defense. Below are the most trusted solutions for common immune-related concerns, organized by specific needs and supported by both customer-reported experiences and science-informed insights.

Frequent Illness and Immune Weakness

A weakened immune system can leave the body more susceptible to recurring colds, respiratory infections, and extended recovery times. Supporting immune function may help reduce the frequency of illness and promote faster, more complete recovery.

Top Solutions for Frequent Infections

Astragalus (67%) – Customers report fewer sick days and a stronger sense of immune resilience. Scientific Support: Astragalus enhances white blood cell function, supporting the body's natural defense against bacteria and viruses.

Oregano Oil (44%) – Many users find it helpful for reducing the frequency of infections and supporting quicker recovery. Scientific Support: Oregano oil contains carvacrol and thymol, compounds with natural antimicrobial and antiviral properties.

Elderberry (43%) – Users frequently note shorter duration and milder symptoms during cold and flu season. Scientific Support: Elderberry is rich in anthocyanins, which help modulate immune response and reduce viral replication.

Turkey Tail (30%) – Many report improved immune resilience during seasonal transitions. Scientific Support: Turkey Tail contains polysaccharide-K (PSK), which supports immune activation and enhances overall immune function.

Reishi (30%) – Users often mention fewer infections and improved overall immunity. Scientific Support: Reishi mushrooms provide beta-glucans, which influence immune signaling and promote white blood cell activity.

Agarikon (55%) – Many users find Agarikon beneficial during times of heightened exposure to cold and flu viruses. Scientific Support: Agarikon shows both antiviral and antimicrobial activity, supporting general immune health.

Thymus (50%) – Users report fewer infections and faster recovery when using thymus-based supplements. Scientific Support: Thymus extracts help support T-cell development, a key part of adaptive immune defense.

Vitamin D (41%) – Many find that consistent use of vitamin D is linked to fewer seasonal illnesses. Scientific Support: Vitamin D is involved in activating immune cells and maintaining immune balance.

Summary Table: Frequent Illness and Immune Weakness

Therapy	Solution	Details
Herbal Therapy	Astragalus	67% of users report fewer sick days; enhances immune response.
Herbal Therapy	Oregano Oil	44% of users find it helps prevent infections; contains antimicrobial compounds.
Herbal Therapy	Elderberry	43% of users report faster recovery; supports immune resilience.
Mushroom Therapy	Turkey Tail	30% of users report better immune function; contains immune-activating polysaccharides.
Mushroom Therapy	Reishi	30% of users report improved immunity; beta-glucans modulate immune response.
Mushroom Therapy	Agarikon	55% of users report fewer colds; antiviral and antimicrobial benefits.
Animal Organ Therapy	Thymus	50% of users report fewer infections; supports T-cell function.
HOPED Protocol	Vitamin D	41% of users report better immunity; essential for immune cell activation.

To learn what research and real-world experience reveal about each of these solutions, and which one might be a good fit for you, see the corresponding therapy books in The Medicine-Free, Illness-Free Series.

Immune Resilience and Cellular Defense

The immune system plays a vital role not only in defending against infections but also in identifying and addressing abnormal cells before they can disrupt healthy function. When immune surveillance is weakened, the body may be less equipped to detect and respond to cellular irregularities, increasing long-term health risks. This makes immune-supportive strategies an important part of promoting cellular integrity and long-term resilience.

Top Solutions for Immune Resilience and Cellular Defense

Turkey Tail (40%) – Many users take Turkey Tail to support immune strength during intensive health challenges. Scientific Support: Turkey Tail contains polysaccharide-K (PSK), a compound that supports immune activity and has been used in clinical settings as an immune-enhancing adjunct.

Shiitake (25%) – Customers report feeling more resilient when incorporating Shiitake alongside conventional therapies. Scientific Support: Shiitake mushrooms provide lentinan, a beta-glucan that supports immune activity and may help defend against abnormal cell growth.

Maitake (23%) – Users find Maitake helpful for supporting prostate and cellular health. Scientific Support: Maitake D-fraction has been studied for its ability to support immune modulation and inhibit abnormal cellular proliferation.

Chaga (20%) – Customers often report increased vitality and immune strength when using Chaga. Scientific Support: Chaga is high in antioxidants, which help reduce oxidative stress, a key factor in immune regulation and cellular defense.

Thymus (50%) – Users report stronger immune response and recovery during health challenges. Scientific Support: Thymus extracts help regulate immune cell activity and support immune surveillance mechanisms

Summary Table: Immune Resilience and Cellular Defense

Therapy	Solution	Details
Mushroom Therapy	Turkey Tail	40% of users take it for immune support during treatment; contains PSK, an immune-enhancing polysaccharide.
Mushroom Therapy	Shiitake	25% of users report improved resilience; contains lentinan, which supports immune function.
Mushroom Therapy	Maitake	23% of users report benefits for prostate and cellular health; Maitake D-fraction supports immune modulation.
Mushroom Therapy	Chaga	20% of users report stronger immune resilience; rich in antioxidants that reduce oxidative stress.
Animal Organ Therapy	Thymus	50% of users report improved immune response; supports T-cell function and immune surveillance.

To learn what research and real-world experience reveal about each of these solutions, and which one might be a good fit for you, see the corresponding therapy books in The Medicine-Free, Illness-Free Series.

Environmental or Food Sensitivity

Sensitivities to environmental triggers or certain foods occur when the immune system becomes overreactive to otherwise harmless substances such as pollen, dust, or food-based proteins. This heightened immune response may contribute to respiratory challenges (such as seasonal discomfort) or food-related sensitivities (such as histamine intolerance). The right natural support may help regulate immune responses, easing sensitivity symptoms while maintaining overall immune function.

Top Solutions for Immune Sensitivities and Overreaction

Thymus (28%) – Users report fewer seasonal flare-ups and improved respiratory comfort. Scientific Support: Thymus peptides help support immune balance by regulating immune cell activity and reducing unnecessary inflammation.

Kidney (26%) – Many customers note improved tolerance to food triggers and histamine-rich foods. Scientific Support: Kidney tissue naturally contains diamine oxidase (DAO), an enzyme involved in breaking down histamine and supporting healthy immune response to dietary antigens.

Summary Table: Immune Sensitivities and Overreaction

Therapy	Solution	Details
Animal Organ Therapy	Thymus	28% of users report fewer allergy symptoms; helps regulate immune response to reduce inflammation.
Animal Organ Therapy	Kidney	26% of users report reduced food-related sensitivities; provides DAO enzymes to break down excess histamine.

To learn what research and real-world experience reveal about each of these solutions, and which one might be a good fit for you, see the corresponding therapy books in The Medicine-Free, Illness-Free Series.

Cognitive Health

Cognitive health is the foundation of our ability to think clearly, remember important information, and stay mentally sharp throughout life. Whether it involves recalling details, maintaining focus during demanding tasks, or supporting long-term brain performance, healthy cognitive function is essential for overall well-being. However, today's fast-paced lifestyles, marked by chronic stress, poor nutrition, environmental toxin exposure, and insufficient sleep, can place significant strain on the brain.

Fortunately, the brain is a highly adaptable organ with the ability to repair, reorganize, and regenerate when given the right support. While lifestyle factors such as restorative sleep, mental engagement, and nutrient-rich foods are essential, targeted natural therapies can further help optimize mental performance and cognitive resilience. This section outlines science-informed solutions for common concerns including memory decline, reduced focus, mental fatigue, attention challenges, and age-related cognitive changes.

By incorporating select herbs, mushrooms, organ extracts, amino acids, and key nutrients, you can help nourish brain function, support healthy neurological signaling, and promote mental clarity. Each solution presented here is supported by real-world customer experience and scientific insight, offering a practical path to improving cognitive performance in everyday life.

Memory and Mental Clarity

Memory concerns, whether occasional forgetfulness or difficulty retaining new information, can affect individuals at any stage of life, especially as they age. While mild lapses are common, ongoing memory challenges may point to deeper cognitive strain. Supporting brain function with carefully selected herbs, mushrooms, organ supplements, amino acids, and targeted nutrients may help strengthen recall, enhance learning, and reduce mental fatigue.

Top Solutions for Memory Support

Bacopa (35% Memory Enhancement, 27% Cognitive Function) – Users report better recall, stronger retention, and improved cognitive processing. Scientific Support: Bacopa monnieri has been shown to enhance memory performance and support mental clarity in multiple studies.

Ginkgo (60%) – Many users describe sharper mental clarity and improved memory retention. Scientific Support: Ginkgo biloba supports cerebral blood flow, which may benefit memory and cognitive function.

Lion's Mane (40%) – Frequently mentioned for improving memory and information retention. Scientific Support: Lion's Mane stimulates nerve growth factor (NGF), supporting neuronal growth and cognitive resilience.

Brain (13%) – Some users report improvement in both short- and long-term memory. Scientific Support: Brain extracts contain neuropeptides that support synaptic plasticity and the formation of memory pathways.

Serine (31%) – Users note better memory retention and more consistent recall. Scientific Support: Serine contributes to neurotransmitter synthesis and plays a key role in maintaining cognitive performance.

Fish Eggs (22%) – Many users report enhanced memory and clearer thinking. Scientific Support: Fish eggs contain omega-3 fatty acids and phospholipids that support brain structure and neuronal communication.

Summary Table: Memory Support Solutions

Therapy	Solution	Details
Herbal Therapy	Bacopa	35% of users report better memory; enhances recall and retention.
Herbal Therapy	Ginkgo	60% of users note sharper mental clarity; increases blood flow to the brain.
Mushroom Therapy	Lion's Mane	40% of users report improved memory; stimulates NGF to support cognition.
Animal Organ Therapy	Brain	13% of users see better recall; neuropeptides enhance memory formation.
Animal Organ Therapy	Fish Eggs	22% of users report enhanced memory. Omega-3 for brain health.
Amino Acid Therapy	Serine	31% of users experience improved retention; supports neurotransmitter synthesis.

To learn what research and real-world experience reveal about each of these solutions, and which one might be a good fit for you, see the corresponding therapy books in The Medicine-Free, Illness-Free Series.

Cognitive Performance Support

Cognitive decline refers to the gradual reduction in mental sharpness that often accompanies aging. While some cognitive slowing is expected over time, chronic inflammation, oxidative stress, and lifestyle challenges may accelerate this process and place additional strain on brain function. Supporting cognitive performance with targeted natural solutions can help maintain clarity, improve mental agility, and protect long-term brain health.

Top Solutions for Cognitive Aging and Performance

Lion's Mane (40%) – Users report greater cognitive longevity and reduced mental decline. Scientific Support: Lion's Mane promotes nerve regeneration and supports the brain's ability to adapt and maintain function with age.

Ginkgo (60%) – Many users experience enhanced mental clarity and fewer signs of age-related decline. Scientific Support: Ginkgo supports cerebral blood circulation and reduces oxidative stress in brain tissue.

Brain (10%) – Users describe sharper thinking and more efficient mental processing. Scientific Support: Brain extracts provide fats and peptides that aid neurotransmission and overall brain signaling.

Fish Oil (13%) – Customers report clearer thinking and better concentration. Scientific Support: Omega-3 fatty acids such as DHA and EPA nourish neuronal membranes and help counter oxidative damage.

Vitamin D (13%) – Users experience improved mental alertness and balanced mood. Scientific Support: Vitamin D influences neurotransmitter pathways through its receptors in brain tissue, supporting cognitive resilience.

Summary Table: Cognitive Performance and Aging Support

Therapy	Solution	Details
Mushroom Therapy	Lion's Mane	40% of users report sharper cognitive function; supports NGF synthesis.
Herbal Therapy	Ginkgo	60% of users see reduced cognitive decline; improves blood circulation.
Animal Organ Therapy	Brain	10% of users experience better mental performance; supports neurotransmission.
HOPED Protocol	Fish Oil	13% of users report better focus; DHA/EPA nourish brain cells.
HOPED Protocol	Vitamin D	13% of users note improved mood and cognitive sharpness.

To learn what research and real-world experience reveal about each of these solutions, and which one might be a good fit for you, see the corresponding therapy books in The Medicine-Free, Illness-Free Series.

Focus and Attention Support

Difficulty concentrating, mental fatigue, and short attention spans can disrupt productivity, decision-making, and daily performance. Whether these challenges stem from stress, poor sleep, or neurological imbalances, targeted natural support may help improve focus, sustain attention, and restore mental clarity throughout the day.

Top Solutions for Focus and Attention

Lion's Mane (30%) – Users report reduced brain fog and improved concentration. Scientific Support: Lion's Mane supports mental clarity and focus through its effects on nerve growth factor (NGF).

Rhodiola (26%) – Many find it enhances focus and cognitive performance during stressful periods. Scientific Support: Rhodiola is an adaptogen that promotes mental stamina and sustained attention.

Brain (25%) – Customers often describe sharper focus and improved productivity. Scientific Support: Brain-derived phospholipids support neurotransmission and cognitive signaling.

Tyrosine (28%) – Reported to increase alertness and focus. Scientific Support: Tyrosine is a precursor to dopamine, supporting motivation and mental clarity.

Bacopa (18%) – Users experience improved attention span and task completion. Scientific Support: Bacopa supports cognitive processing speed and attention regulation.

Cordyceps (10%) – Described by users as helpful for sustaining concentration and mental energy. Scientific Support: Cordyceps has been linked to improved oxygen utilization and brain function under stress.

Summary Table: Focus and Attention Support Solutions

Therapy	Solution	Details
Herbal Therapy	Bacopa	18% of users report better focus; enhances attention span.
Mushroom Therapy	Lion's Mane	30% of users report better concentration; reduces brain fog.

Therapy	Solution	Details
Herbal Therapy	Rhodiola	26% of users experience improved cognitive function; enhances mental clarity.
Animal Organ Therapy	Brain	25% of users note better focus; phospholipids support cognition.
Amino Acid Therapy	Tyrosine	28% of users report better attention span; supports dopamine production.
Mushroom Therapy	Cordyceps	10% of users report better focus and clarity; supports improved cognitive function.

To learn what research and real-world experience reveal about each of these solutions, and which one might be a good fit for you, see the corresponding therapy books in The Medicine-Free, Illness-Free Series.

Overstimulation and Cognitive Balance

Overstimulation, impulsivity, and attention challenges can affect both children and adults, often impacting learning, productivity, and emotional well-being. These patterns are commonly associated with neurodevelopmental conditions and may also arise from modern lifestyle stressors, environmental exposures, or imbalances in neurotransmitter activity. While conventional treatments often rely on stimulants, natural solutions offer supportive options that promote focus, emotional regulation, and cognitive balance without the common side effects.

Select herbs, mushrooms, amino acids, and detox protocols may help enhance neurotransmitter balance, support brain function, and reduce the effects of mental overstimulation. These approaches work by promoting dopamine and norepinephrine activity, reducing oxidative stress, and sustaining healthy cognitive energy and control.

Top Solutions for Focus and Impulse Regulation

Bacopa (18%) – Users frequently report improved attention span, focus, and mental processing. Scientific Support: Bacopa monnieri has been shown to support dopamine signaling and cognitive performance, making it a useful option for attention and regulation support.

Lion's Mane (30%) – Many individuals note improved concentration and reduced mental fatigue. Scientific Support: Lion's Mane promotes nerve growth factor (NGF) activity, which supports neural development and cognitive flexibility.

Tyrosine (28%) – Commonly used to enhance alertness and maintain focus. Scientific Support: Tyrosine serves as a precursor to dopamine and norepinephrine, which are critical for attention, motivation, and executive function.

Phenylalanine (16%) – Reported to help with sustained focus and mental sharpness. Scientific Support: Phenylalanine converts into tyrosine and contributes to healthy neurotransmitter production, supporting cognitive regulation.

Heavy Metal Detox for Kids (30%) – Parents often observe better speech, behavior, and focus following gentle detox protocols. Scientific Support: Reducing heavy metal exposure may alleviate neurotoxic burden, which has been linked to developmental and cognitive challenges.

Quick-Reference Table: Focus, Impulse and Overstimulation Support

Therapy	Solution	Details
Herbal Therapy	Bacopa	18% of users report enhanced focus; supports dopamine function for better attention.
Mushroom Therapy	Lion's Mane	30% of users experience improved concentration and mental energy; promotes nerve growth factor (NGF).
Amino Acid Therapy	Tyrosine	28% of users feel more alert and mentally sharp; precursor to dopamine and norepinephrine.
Amino Acid Therapy	Phenylalanine	16% of users report better mental clarity and impulse control; supports dopamine synthesis.
Detox Therapy	Heavy Metal Detox for Kids	30% of parents note improved cognitive behavior; detoxing heavy metals may reduce neurotoxicity.

To learn what research and real-world experience reveal about each of these solutions, and which one might be a good fit for you, see the corresponding therapy books in The Medicine-Free, Illness-Free Series.

Age-Related Cognitive Challenges

Age-related cognitive decline may involve changes in memory, attention, and executive function, and in more severe cases, may contribute to neurodegenerative conditions. These challenges are often associated with the buildup of oxidative stress, inflammation, and impaired communication between neurons. While conventional medicine focuses on symptom management, natural therapies may help support brain plasticity, protect neurons, and maintain mental clarity during aging.

Many individuals who want to protect long-term brain health or support a loved one experiencing cognitive changes turn to natural solutions that promote memory retention, focus, and neurological resilience.

Top Solutions for Aging Cognitive Support

Lion's Mane (40%) – Many users report improved memory, sharper recall, and cognitive steadiness with regular use. Scientific Support: Lion's Mane stimulates nerve growth factor (NGF), which supports neural regeneration and long-term brain health.

Bacopa (35%) – Users commonly experience better recall and decreased forgetfulness. Scientific Support: Bacopa monnieri helps support acetylcholine activity, a key neurotransmitter involved in learning and memory.

Ginkgo (60%) – Frequently reported to enhance mental alertness and protect brain function. Scientific Support: Ginkgo biloba improves blood circulation in the brain and helps reduce oxidative stress that may affect neurons.

Brain (13%) – Users describe improvements in memory resilience and mental clarity. Scientific Support: Brain peptides contain phospholipids and neurotrophic compounds that help preserve synaptic function and support cognitive adaptation.

Fish Eggs (22%) – Many users report better memory sharpness and reduced signs of cognitive slowdown. Scientific Support: Fish eggs supply DHA, EPA, and phospholipids, all of which support neuronal membrane health and brain longevity.

Fish Oil (13%) – Users often experience more consistent cognitive performance. Scientific Support: Omega-3 fatty acids in fish oil help maintain healthy neuron membranes and reduce brain inflammation associated with aging.

Quick-Reference Table: Age-Related Cognitive Support

Therapy	Solution	Details
Mushroom Therapy	Lion's Mane	40% of users report better memory and recall; stimulates nerve growth factor (NGF).
Herbal Therapy	Bacopa	35% of users experience improved memory retention; supports acetylcholine function for learning.
Herbal Therapy	Ginkgo	60% of users find better mental clarity; increases brain circulation and reduces oxidative stress.
Animal Organ Therapy	Brain	13% of users report enhanced cognitive function; provides neurotrophic factors that protect neurons.
HOPED Protocol	Fish Eggs	22% of users note better cognitive sharpness; Omega-3s support brain longevity.
HOPED Protocol	Fish Oil	13% of users experience improved mental stability; DHA/EPA protect neuronal function.

To learn what research and real-world experience reveal about each of these solutions, and which one might be a good fit for you, see

the corresponding therapy books in The Medicine-Free, Illness-Free Series.

Digestive Health

Your digestive system plays a foundational role in maintaining overall health and vitality. It is responsible for breaking down the food you eat, absorbing nutrients, eliminating waste, and supporting immune balance. When digestive function is working efficiently, you are more likely to feel energized, nourished, and in balance. However, digestive discomfort is increasingly common today, often linked to chronic stress, heavily processed diets, medication overuse, environmental exposures, and sedentary habits.

Challenges such as acid reflux, irregularity, indigestion, gut permeability, and inflammation-related bowel issues can significantly interfere with daily life. These imbalances may lead to bloating, abdominal pain, fatigue, nutrient deficiencies, and increased systemic inflammation. Fortunately, a variety of natural therapies offer gentle and effective support by addressing the underlying causes of digestive distress, including inflammation, enzyme insufficiency, microbial imbalances, and compromised gut lining integrity.

Below, you'll find carefully selected natural solutions organized by digestive concern. These recommendations are based on real-world customer experience and scientific research, helping you explore practical ways to support healthy digestion and regain lasting comfort and vitality.

Acid Reflux and Balance

Gastroesophageal Reflux Disease (GERD), commonly referred to as acid reflux, occurs when stomach acid moves backward into the esophagus. This can lead to heartburn, irritation, inflammation, and over time, damage to the esophageal lining. If not addressed, chronic reflux may contribute to conditions such as esophagitis and Barrett's esophagus.

Laryngopharyngeal Reflux (LPR), sometimes called silent reflux, is a related issue in which stomach acid travels even higher into the throat, reaching the larynx and pharynx. LPR often does not cause heartburn, but may present as chronic throat irritation, hoarseness, postnasal drip, persistent cough, or difficulty swallowing.

Both GERD and LPR are associated with disruptions in stomach acid balance and incomplete digestion. Natural therapies may help restore proper acidity, support more complete digestion, and protect sensitive tissues from acid-related damage.

Top Solutions for Acid Reflux and Silent Reflux (LPR) Support

DGL Licorice (44%) – Users report quick relief from heartburn and throat irritation. Scientific Support: DGL stimulates mucus production, helping to coat and protect the esophagus and gastrointestinal lining.

Betaine HCL (30%) – Many individuals find it helps improve digestion and reduce reflux symptoms. Scientific Support: Betaine HCL supports optimal stomach acid levels, which helps prevent regurgitation and supports nutrient breakdown.

Pancreas (27%) – Users note reduced digestive discomfort and more efficient digestion. Scientific Support: Pancreatic enzymes aid in breaking down fats, proteins, and carbohydrates, helping to ease gastric stress and reduce pressure on the stomach.

Summary Table: Acid Reflux and Silent Reflux Support

Therapy	Solution	Details
Herbal Therapy	DGL Licorice	44% of users report relief from reflux; stimulates mucus to protect tissue.
HOPED Protocol	Betaine HCL	30% of users report improved digestion; restores optimal stomach acidity.
Animal Organ Therapy	Pancreas	27% of users report reduced gastric distress; provides digestive enzyme support.

To learn what research and real-world experience reveal about each of these solutions, and which one might be a good fit for you, see the corresponding therapy books in The Medicine-Free, Illness-Free Series.

Bloating, Gas, and Irregularity

Digestive discomfort marked by bloating, gas, and unpredictable bowel patterns is a common concern for many individuals. These symptoms are often associated with gut sensitivity, microbial imbalance, irregular motility, and poor nutrient absorption. Factors such as stress, dietary triggers, and a disrupted gut-brain connection may also contribute to recurring digestive upset.

Natural therapies may help restore microbial balance, support healthy motility, strengthen the intestinal lining, and reduce discomfort. These approaches focus on improving how the gut functions, rather than simply masking symptoms.

Top Solutions for Digestive Irregularity and Bloating

Gut Probiotics (42%) – Users report reduced bloating, better bowel regularity, and improved digestive comfort. Scientific Support:

Beneficial bacteria help regulate digestion, support gut motility, and promote immune balance.

Glutamine (43%) – Many experience relief from abdominal discomfort and improved intestinal integrity. Scientific Support: Glutamine helps repair the gut lining and supports the healing of inflamed intestinal tissues.

Pancreatin (28%) – Frequently used to relieve post-meal bloating and cramping. Scientific Support: Pancreatin supplies digestive enzymes that enhance nutrient breakdown and ease gastric stress.

Turkey Tail Mushroom (15%) – Users note improved gut health and reduced irregularity. Scientific Support: Turkey Tail promotes beneficial bacteria in the gut, supporting balanced digestion and microbial harmony.

Summary Table: Bloating, Gas, and Irregularity Support

Therapy	Solution	Details
HOPED Protocol	Gut Probiotics	42% of users report balanced microbiome and symptom relief.
Amino Acid Therapy	Glutamine	43% of users report improved gut comfort; helps repair intestinal lining.
HOPED Protocol	Pancreatin	28% of users note reduced bloating; enhances digestion after meals.
Mushroom Therapy	Turkey Tail	15% of users report better digestion; supports microbial balance.

To learn what research and real-world experience reveal about each of these solutions, and which one might be a good fit for you, see the corresponding therapy books in The Medicine-Free, Illness-Free Series.

Constipation Support

Chronic constipation and irregular bowel movements can lead to significant discomfort, abdominal bloating, toxin buildup, and reduced nutrient absorption. Common contributing factors include low fiber intake, inadequate hydration, a sedentary lifestyle, and gut flora imbalance. Natural therapies can support digestive motility, encourage regular elimination, and help maintain overall digestive comfort.

Top Solutions for Constipation and Irregularity

Psyllium Husk (50%) – Users report dramatic improvement in regularity and overall digestive ease. Scientific Support: Psyllium is rich in soluble fiber, which adds bulk to stool and promotes consistent bowel movements.

Colon Detox (24%) – Customers experience gentler, more consistent elimination and less bloating. Scientific Support: Colon detox formulations may include herbs and fibers that stimulate motility and support natural cleansing of the digestive tract.

Summary Table: Constipation Support

Therapy	Solution	Details
HOPED Protocol	Psyllium Husk	50% of users report improved regularity; fiber promotes elimination.
Detox Therapy	Colon Detox	24% of users experience easier bowel movements; supports colon health.

To learn what research and real-world experience reveal about each of these solutions, and which one might be a good fit for you, see

the corresponding therapy books in The Medicine-Free, Illness-Free Series.

Indigestion and Digestive Discomfort

Indigestion, also known as dyspepsia, commonly leads to bloating, stomach discomfort, early fullness, nausea, and excess gas following meals. These symptoms may stem from inadequate digestive enzymes, microbial imbalance, suboptimal eating habits, or low-grade inflammation. Natural therapies can help improve digestive function, reduce discomfort, and support more efficient nutrient breakdown.

Top Solutions for Indigestion

Pancreatin (64%) – Many users report noticeable relief from bloating and heaviness after meals. Scientific Support: Pancreatin provides key digestive enzymes like amylase, protease, and lipase, which support effective food breakdown and absorption.

Vegan Enzymes (50%) – Users frequently note better digestion of fats, carbohydrates, and proteins. Scientific Support: Plant-based enzymes support digestive efficiency and help reduce post-meal bloating and discomfort.

Pancreas (65%) – Many individuals experience reduced indigestion and improved nutrient assimilation. Scientific Support: Pancreatic extracts support natural enzyme production, enhance breakdown of macronutrients, and promote balanced digestion.

Betaine HCL (45%) – Users report improved protein digestion and reduced digestive sluggishness. Scientific Support: Betaine HCL helps restore optimal stomach acid levels, supporting nutrient breakdown and microbial balance.

DGL Licorice (28%) – Frequently used to ease mild stomach discomfort and soothe the gut lining. Scientific Support: DGL supports mucosal healing and helps reduce inflammation in the digestive tract.

Oregano Oil (25%) – Users find relief from bloating and discomfort, especially after meals. Scientific Support: Oregano oil has antimicrobial effects that help balance gut flora and support healthy digestion.

Summary Table: Indigestion and Digestive Support

Therapy	Solution	Details
HOPED Protocol	Pancreatin	64% of users report relief from indigestion; provides key digestive enzymes.
HOPED Protocol	Vegan Enzymes	50% of users experience better digestion; plant enzymes reduce bloating.
Animal Organ Therapy	Pancreas	65% of users report less discomfort; supports pancreatic enzyme production.
HOPED Protocol	Betaine HCL	45% of users improve protein digestion; supports proper stomach acid levels.
Herbal Therapy	DGL Licorice	28% of users feel stomach relief; promotes mucosal healing.
Herbal Therapy	Oregano Oil	25% of users note better digestion; balances gut flora.

To learn what research and real-world experience reveal about each of these solutions, and which one might be a good fit for you, see the corresponding therapy books in The Medicine-Free, Illness-Free Series.

Gut Integrity and Barrier Support

The intestinal lining serves as a critical barrier between your digestive tract and the rest of your body. When this barrier becomes overly permeable, a condition often referred to as "leaky gut," it may allow unwanted substances such as toxins, microbes, and partially digested food particles to enter the bloodstream. This increased permeability can contribute to inflammation, nutrient malabsorption, food sensitivities, and broader immune system imbalances.

Natural therapies may help restore gut lining integrity, reduce permeability, and support a balanced microbiome. By strengthening this protective barrier, these approaches can contribute to improved digestion, immune regulation, and overall health.

Top Solutions for Gut Barrier Support

Candida & Yeast Detox (69%) – Many users report reduced bloating, improved digestion, and more balanced gut flora. Scientific Support: This approach helps rebalance the microbiota and reduce inflammation associated with microbial overgrowth.

Colostrum (25%) – Users experience greater digestive comfort and improved gut lining function. Scientific Support: Colostrum contains immunoglobulins and growth factors that support gut tissue repair and barrier strength.

Glutamine (13%) – Frequently used to improve gut barrier function and reduce digestive irritation. Scientific Support: Glutamine plays a key role in rebuilding intestinal cells and maintaining a healthy mucosal lining.

Summary Table: Gut Integrity and Barrier Support

Therapy	Solution	Details
Detox Therapy	Candida & Yeast Detox	69% of users report improved gut flora and reduced inflammation; supports microbial balance.
Animal Organ Therapy	Colostrum	25% of users report stronger gut lining; supports mucosal repair.
Amino Acid Therapy	Glutamine	13% of users report improved barrier function; restores intestinal integrity.

To learn what research and real-world experience reveal about each of these solutions, and which one might be a good fit for you, see the corresponding therapy books in The Medicine-Free, Illness-Free Series.

Digestive Inflammation and Resilience

Digestive inflammation can significantly affect quality of life, especially in individuals experiencing chronic symptoms such as abdominal pain, bloating, irregular bowel movements, nutrient malabsorption, and fatigue. These symptoms are often associated with imbalances in the gut microbiome, impaired enzyme production, or a compromised intestinal lining. While chronic inflammatory conditions like Crohn's disease and ulcerative colitis involve more complex medical care, natural therapies may offer supportive benefits by helping reduce inflammation, restore microbial balance, support mucosal repair, and promote better nutrient absorption.

Top Solutions for Digestive Inflammation and Resilience

Parasite Detox (57%) – Many users report less bloating, reduced discomfort, and improved gut balance. Scientific Support: Parasite-cleansing protocols may help reduce microbial burden and gastrointestinal inflammation, supporting a healthier digestive environment.

Pancreas (20%) – Users describe improved digestion and reduced digestive irritation. Scientific Support: Pancreatic extracts supply key enzymes that support digestion and help reduce stress on the gastrointestinal lining.

Colostrum (12%) – Reported to help with gut recovery and improved nutrient utilization. Scientific Support: Colostrum provides growth factors and immunoglobulins that support healing of the intestinal lining and improve absorption.

Summary Table: Digestive Inflammation and Resilience

Therapy	Solution	Details
Detox Therapy	Parasite Detox	57% of users report less inflammation and discomfort; supports microbial balance.
Animal Organ Therapy	Pancreas	20% of users report improved digestion; supports enzyme function and reduces irritation.
Animal Organ Therapy	Colostrum	12% of users report better gut resilience; supports mucosal repair and nutrient uptake.

To learn what research and real-world experience reveal about each of these solutions, and which one might be a good fit for you, see the corresponding therapy books in The Medicine-Free, Illness-Free Series.

Reproductive and Hormonal Support

The reproductive system plays a foundational role in overall well-being, influencing hormonal balance, sexual function, fertility, and emotional regulation. Healthy reproductive function supports the proper production and regulation of key hormones such as testosterone, estrogen, and progesterone. These hormones contribute to libido, menstrual cycle regularity, sperm and egg quality, mood stability, energy, and overall vitality.

However, modern stressors, including emotional strain, poor diet, aging, environmental toxins, and endocrine-disrupting chemicals, can interfere with reproductive health. Many individuals experience symptoms such as low libido, erectile challenges, irregular menstrual cycles, hormonal imbalances, and fertility concerns. These disruptions may also affect emotional resilience, energy levels, and intimacy.

While conventional options may involve hormone replacement therapy, medications, or invasive procedures, natural therapies offer supportive alternatives that work with the body's own rhythms. These approaches focus on restoring hormonal balance, improving circulation, supporting organ function, and enhancing nutrient availability, all of which contribute to reproductive health and vitality.

Below are some of the most widely used natural solutions for reproductive and hormonal concerns. Each therapy is supported by scientific research and real-world user feedback, offering an integrative path toward improved reproductive wellness.

Low Libido and Sexual Vitality Support

Sexual desire and performance are closely connected to overall physical, emotional, and hormonal well-being. When libido decreases or erectile function becomes impaired, it may signal underlying issues such as hormonal imbalance, reduced circulation, chronic stress, or nutrient deficiencies. Testosterone plays a key role in supporting sexual drive for both men and women, while healthy blood flow and nitric oxide production are essential for erectile function in men. Elevated cortisol levels from stress can suppress reproductive hormones, while diet and lifestyle factors may also contribute to low energy and poor circulation.

Natural therapies may help address the root causes of these concerns by promoting testosterone balance, enhancing blood flow, increasing nitric oxide levels, and reducing stress. Many of these remedies have long-standing traditional use and are now supported by scientific studies for their role in supporting sexual vitality.

Top Solutions for Sexual Function and Desire

Maca (20%) – Users report increased libido, stamina, and improved performance. Scientific Support: Traditionally used in Peru, maca supports hormonal balance and energy, promoting sexual well-being in both men and women.

Ginseng (15%) – Often used to improve erectile strength and male libido. Scientific Support: Ginseng enhances nitric oxide production, leading to better circulation and firmer erections.

Ashwagandha (13%) – Frequently mentioned for restoring desire and physical endurance. Scientific Support: Ashwagandha reduces cortisol levels and supports healthy hormone levels, improving arousal and resilience.

Arginine (19%) – Users note stronger and more sustained erections. Scientific Support: Arginine is a precursor to nitric oxide, which enhances blood flow and vascular function.

D-Aspartic Acid (13%) – Many men report increased testosterone and improved sperm quality. Scientific Support: DAA stimulates the release of hormones involved in testosterone production.

Shilajit (10%) – Associated with improved male vitality and overall reproductive support. Scientific Support: Shilajit provides minerals and fulvic acid, helping to support hormone regulation and energy.

Summary Table: Low Libido and Erectile Function Support

Therapy	Solution	Details
Herbal Therapy	Maca	20% of users report increased libido and performance; supports stamina and hormone balance.
Herbal Therapy	Ginseng	15% of users report better erectile function; promotes nitric oxide production.
Herbal Therapy	Ashwagandha	13% of users experience improved arousal and endurance; reduces stress hormones.
Amino Acid Therapy	Arginine	19% of users report stronger erections; enhances circulation via nitric oxide.
Amino Acid Therapy	DAA	13% of users report increased testosterone; supports hormonal signaling.
HOPED Protocol	Shilajit	10% of users report greater reproductive vitality; rich in fulvic acid and trace minerals.

To learn what research and real-world experience reveal about each of these solutions, and which one might be a good fit for you, see the corresponding therapy books in The Medicine-Free, Illness-Free Series.

Fertility Support

Fertility is a multifaceted process influenced by hormonal balance, reproductive organ function, egg and sperm quality, and overall physical health. For women, stable levels of estrogen and progesterone are essential for regular ovulation, while men require sufficient testosterone to support healthy sperm production. Factors such as chronic stress, oxidative damage, poor nutrition, and exposure to endocrine-disrupting chemicals can negatively affect fertility and complicate the process of conception.

Natural therapies may help enhance reproductive potential by regulating hormonal activity, improving sperm motility and egg quality, and reducing oxidative stress. These approaches are designed to support the body's natural rhythms and create an internal environment more conducive to conception.

Top Solutions for Fertility Support

Ashwagandha (29%) – Users report more balanced hormones and improved fertility outcomes. Scientific Support: Ashwagandha helps regulate cortisol levels, which in turn supports reproductive hormone balance in both men and women.

Maca (37%) – Often used to support menstrual regularity and hormonal stability. Scientific Support: Maca promotes balanced reproductive hormone levels and supports ovulation, particularly in women experiencing irregular cycles.

Female Organs (9%) – Users report more consistent menstrual cycles and improved reproductive health. Scientific Support: Female organ extracts contain cofactors and nutrients that may support ovarian function and hormone regulation.

Testicles (9%) – Reported to improve male fertility indicators such as sperm motility and vitality. Scientific Support: Testicular extracts provide natural androgen precursors that support testosterone production and sperm quality.

Arginine (19%) – Users frequently note improved reproductive circulation and better sperm health. Scientific Support: Arginine boosts nitric oxide levels, which support healthy blood flow and sperm motility.

D-Aspartic Acid (13%) – Many men report improved testosterone levels and enhanced sperm count. Scientific Support: DAA influences the hypothalamic-pituitary-gonadal axis, stimulating natural testosterone production and reproductive hormone signaling.

Summary Table: Fertility Support

Therapy	Solution	Details
Herbal Therapy	Ashwagandha	29% of users report better hormone balance and fertility support.
Herbal Therapy	Maca	37% of users report improved menstrual cycles and hormone stability.
Animal Organ Therapy	Female Organs	9% of users report more regular cycles; supports ovarian function.
Animal Organ Therapy	Testicles	9% of users report improved male fertility; enhances testosterone.

Therapy	Solution	Details
Amino Acid Therapy	Arginine	19% of users report better sperm motility; improves circulation.
Amino Acid Therapy	DAA	13% of users report increased testosterone; supports sperm production.

To learn what research and real-world experience reveal about each of these solutions, and which one might be a good fit for you, see the corresponding therapy books in The Medicine-Free, Illness-Free Series.

Hormonal Balance

Hormonal imbalances can contribute to a wide range of health concerns, including menstrual irregularities, mood changes, weight fluctuations, fatigue, and low energy. In women, imbalanced estrogen and progesterone levels may lead to severe premenstrual symptoms, ovulatory issues, or menopausal discomfort. In men, lower testosterone may result in decreased motivation, reduced muscle tone, and diminished sexual drive. These hormonal disruptions are often linked to chronic stress, nutrient deficiencies, environmental exposures, or suboptimal adrenal function.

Natural therapies may help support the endocrine system by promoting balance in estrogen, progesterone, and testosterone levels. Unlike synthetic hormone therapies, these approaches are designed to work with the body's own hormonal rhythms, supporting long-term wellness with fewer side effects.

Top Solutions for Hormonal Balance Support

Maca (37%) – Users report more regular menstrual cycles and improved hormonal stability. Scientific Support: Maca supports endocrine regulation and helps balance estrogen and progesterone levels, particularly during hormonal transitions.

Ashwagandha (29%) – Frequently used to ease hormone-related symptoms and restore vitality. Scientific Support: As an adaptogen, Ashwagandha helps lower cortisol and supports adrenal health, contributing to hormonal equilibrium.

Female Organs (23%) – Users describe fewer mood swings and better cycle regularity. Scientific Support: Female organ extracts provide hormone precursors and cofactors that support estrogen and progesterone production and emotional regulation.

Testicles (9%) – Commonly used to support male hormone balance and vitality. Scientific Support: Testicular extracts contain naturally occurring androgens that help maintain testosterone levels in men with age-related or stress-induced decline.

Summary Table: Hormonal Imbalance Support

Therapy	Solution	Details
Herbal Therapy	Maca	37% of users report improved cycle regularity; supports hormone balance.
Herbal Therapy	Ashwagandha	29% of users report reduced hormonal symptoms; supports adrenal and cortisol balance.
Animal Organ Therapy	Female Organs	23% of users report better emotional stability; supports reproductive hormone production.
Animal Organ Therapy	Testicles	9% of users report enhanced testosterone levels; supports male hormone function.

To learn what research and real-world experience reveal about each of these solutions, and which one might be a good fit for you, see the corresponding therapy books in The Medicine-Free, Illness-Free Series.

Lactation Support

Breastfeeding is an important part of early motherhood, offering bonding and nourishment for the baby. However, low or inconsistent milk supply can create stress and frustration for many new mothers. Contributing factors often include hormonal shifts, nutrient depletion, emotional fatigue, and physical exhaustion. Supporting lactation naturally may help enhance milk flow, improve breast milk quality, and restore the mother's overall strength and vitality.

Natural therapies aim to nourish the body, support postpartum hormone balance, and provide essential nutrients that contribute to successful breastfeeding and maternal wellness.

Top Solutions for Lactation Support

Moringa (19%) – Frequently reported to boost milk production and support maternal energy. Scientific Support: Moringa is rich in vitamins, minerals, and amino acids, and has been shown to support prolactin production, the hormone responsible for lactation, while also improving the nutritional quality of breast milk.

Summary Table: Lactation Support:

Therapy	Solution	Details
Herbal Therapy	Moringa	19% of users report increased milk supply; supports maternal nutrition and lactation hormones.

To learn what research and real-world experience reveal about this solution, and whether it might be a good fit for you, see the corresponding therapy books in The Medicine-Free, Illness-Free Series.

Urinary Health

The urinary system is essential for maintaining internal balance by filtering waste, regulating hydration, supporting electrolyte balance, and eliminating toxins. It includes the kidneys, bladder, ureters, and urethra, all working together to preserve metabolic function and overall homeostasis. When functioning properly, the urinary system also contributes to blood pressure regulation, infection defense, and the removal of metabolic byproducts.

Urinary health can be disrupted by various factors, including bacterial overgrowth, inflammation, hormonal changes, prostate enlargement, or reduced kidney function. Common concerns such as urinary tract discomfort, frequent urination, bladder irritation, and mild kidney strain may interfere with daily comfort and long-term well-being.

While conventional treatments like antibiotics and medications are commonly used, natural therapies may offer gentle, supportive alternatives. These therapies focus on promoting healthy urinary flow, reducing inflammation, supporting microbial balance, and enhancing kidney and bladder function. Backed by both traditional use and scientific investigation, these approaches include herbs, functional mushrooms, amino acids, and nutrient-rich organ extracts that help restore balance to the urinary system.

Below are some of the most frequently used and well-reviewed natural solutions for urinary health, categorized by condition and supported by customer-reported experiences and scientific insights.

Urinary Tract Support

Urinary tract infections (UTIs) are among the most common urinary health concerns, affecting millions of people each year. They occur when bacteria, most frequently *Escherichia coli* (E. coli), enter the urinary tract, leading to symptoms such as burning during urination, frequent urges to urinate, bladder discomfort, and, in more serious cases, discomfort that may extend toward the kidneys.

Recurrent UTIs may be associated with bacterial adherence to the bladder lining, hormonal fluctuations, or immune system imbalance. While women are more commonly affected due to anatomical differences, men may also experience UTIs, especially when urinary flow is affected by prostate issues.

Natural therapies aim to reduce the likelihood of bacterial adhesion, support microbial balance, soothe irritation, and help the body flush out unwanted organisms. These approaches are widely used for both prevention and comfort.

Top Solutions for Urinary Tract Health

Cranberry (55%) – Frequently used to reduce the risk of recurring UTIs. Scientific Support: Cranberry is rich in proanthocyanidins, which help prevent E. coli from adhering to the bladder lining.

D-Mannose (55%) – Commonly taken to help clear infections and prevent recurrence. Scientific Support: D-Mannose binds to E. coli and supports its natural elimination through urine.

D-Mannose (18%) – Reported to ease burning and urinary discomfort during active infections. Scientific Support: Clinical studies show that D-Mannose can reduce common UTI symptoms while supporting bacterial clearance.

D-Mannose (13%) – Often used preventively by individuals prone to post-intercourse UTIs. Scientific Support: When taken before or after sexual activity, D-Mannose may reduce the risk of bacterial colonization in the urinary tract.

Cranberry (15%) – Also reported to support kidney comfort and urinary detoxification. Scientific Support: In addition to its anti-adhesive properties, cranberry contains antioxidants that help support kidney and bladder health.

Summary Table: Urinary Tract Support

Therapy	Solution	Details
Herbal Therapy	Cranberry	55% of users report fewer UTIs; prevents bacterial adhesion.
HOPED Protocol	D-Mannose	55% of users report reduced recurrence; binds to E. coli for removal.
HOPED Protocol	D-Mannose	18% of users report symptom relief; eases discomfort during UTIs.
HOPED Protocol	D-Mannose	13% of users report fewer UTIs after intercourse; supports prevention.
Herbal Therapy	Cranberry	15% of users report kidney support; offers anti-inflammatory benefits.

Note: When a single solution appears in multiple lines, Such as D-Mannose, each entry reflects a different user-reported benefit or pattern of use. This format helps illustrate the range of experiences and outcomes observed. For more details on how each solution works and how to use it effectively, see the corresponding therapy book in *The Medicine-Free, Illness-Free Series.*

To learn what research and real-world experience reveal about each of these solutions, and which one might be a good fit for you, see

the corresponding therapy books in The Medicine-Free, Illness-Free Series.

Prostate Function Support

Prostate health plays a central role in urinary function, hormonal balance, and male reproductive wellness. As men grow older, it is common for the prostate gland to enlarge, a condition known as benign prostatic hyperplasia (BPH). This may result in urinary symptoms such as frequent urges, weak flow, incomplete emptying, and increased nighttime urination.

An enlarged prostate can place pressure on the urethra, making it harder to urinate and contributing to ongoing discomfort. Natural therapies may help support prostate function by promoting healthy hormone metabolism, reducing inflammation, and improving urinary flow.

Top Solutions for Prostate Health

Saw Palmetto (53%) – Frequently used to support urinary ease and reduce symptoms of BPH. Scientific Support: Saw Palmetto helps inhibit the conversion of testosterone to dihydrotestosterone (DHT), a hormone associated with prostate enlargement. It is often used to reduce urinary frequency and support urinary flow in aging men.

Maitake (23%) – Reported to support prostate cellular health and recovery. Scientific Support: Maitake contains D-fraction polysaccharides that modulate immune activity and may support healthy prostate cell function. It is often used as part of integrative wellness approaches.

Summary Table: Prostate Health Support

Therapy	Solution	Details
Herbal Therapy	Saw Palmetto	53% of users report improved urinary flow and comfort; supports hormone metabolism.
Mushroom Therapy	Maitake	23% of users report support for prostate health and immune modulation.

To learn what research and real-world experience reveal about each of these solutions, and which one might be a good fit for you, see the corresponding therapy books in The Medicine-Free, Illness-Free Series.

Kidney Function Support

The kidneys are vital for filtering waste from the blood, maintaining fluid balance, and regulating key electrolytes. When kidney function becomes compromised, individuals may experience water retention, fatigue, urinary changes, and increased risk for kidney stones or chronic kidney challenges.

Factors such as chronic stress, excess sodium intake, dehydration, and exposure to environmental toxins can place strain on the kidneys, reducing their efficiency over time. Natural therapies aim to support healthy kidney function, promote detoxification, and reduce oxidative stress to help maintain overall renal health.

Top Solutions for Kidney Health

Kidney (44%) – Frequently used to support healthy urine flow and reduce fluid retention. Scientific Support: Kidney-derived organ supplements deliver tissue-specific nutrients and peptides that support detoxification and kidney regeneration.

Kidney Detox (57%) – Often used to enhance filtration efficiency and ease renal burden. Scientific Support: Herbal blends in kidney detox formulas may help support urinary elimination, reduce inflammation, and protect the kidneys from oxidative damage.

Summary Table: Kidney Health and Detoxification

Therapy	Solution	Details
Animal Organ Therapy	Kidney	44% of users report improved kidney function and fluid balance; supports detoxification.
Detox Therapy	Kidney Detox	57% of users report better filtration and comfort; supports urinary and renal health.

To learn what research and real-world experience reveal about each of these solutions, and which one might be a good fit for you, see the corresponding therapy books in The Medicine-Free, Illness-Free Series.

Stress and Emotional Well-being

Stress is a natural biological response that allows the body to adapt to physical, mental, or emotional challenges. In short bursts, it can be motivating and protective. However, when stress becomes chronic or prolonged, it can disrupt nearly every aspect of health, including mood, energy, sleep, digestion, and immune function.

The body's stress response is regulated by the hypothalamic-pituitary-adrenal (HPA) axis and key neurotransmitters such as dopamine, serotonin, and GABA. When this system becomes dysregulated due to persistent stress, trauma, or lifestyle imbalances, individuals may experience symptoms such as fatigue, anxiety, low mood, emotional reactivity, difficulty focusing, and physical tension.

Long-term stress may also contribute to adrenal strain, altered hormone signaling, immune suppression, and increased risk of cardiovascular or metabolic dysfunction. While prescription medications are commonly used to manage anxiety and depression, natural therapies offer supportive alternatives that are non-habit forming and work with the body's natural chemistry.

By strengthening the stress response system, supporting adrenal function, and helping regulate mood-related neurotransmitters, natural therapies may promote emotional stability, mental clarity, and overall resilience.

Chronic Stress Support

Chronic stress occurs when the body's stress response remains continuously activated, often due to persistent mental, emotional, or physical strain. Over time, this ongoing activation may lead to elevated cortisol levels, adrenal fatigue, and dysregulation of the nervous system. Prolonged stress can weaken immunity, impair digestion, disrupt sleep and metabolism, and contribute to emotional exhaustion, burnout, anxiety, or low mood.

Natural therapies for chronic stress aim to support the body's adaptation process by regulating cortisol, restoring adrenal balance, and improving stress resilience. These approaches include adaptogenic herbs, targeted nutrients, organ extracts, and grounding practices that help the body recover and build long-term capacity for handling stress.

Top Solutions to Support Chronic Stress

Ashwagandha (30%) – Commonly reported to reduce feelings of overwhelm and mental tension. Scientific Support: Ashwagandha has been shown to lower cortisol levels and support overall stress regulation.

Licorice (24%) – Frequently used to support adrenal health and energy during long-term stress. Scientific Support: Licorice helps sustain cortisol levels and supports adrenal gland function.

Rhodiola (22%) – Used to maintain energy and mental clarity during stress. Scientific Support: Rhodiola improves endurance and reduces physical and mental fatigue under pressure.

Reishi (20%) – Valued for its calming, restorative properties. Scientific Support: Reishi supports nervous system balance and may help modulate the stress response.

GABA (20%) – Users report a sense of relaxation and less tension during stressful periods. Scientific Support: GABA is an inhibitory neurotransmitter that promotes calm by reducing neural overstimulation.

Shilajit (25%) – Frequently reported to improve clarity, stamina, and stress resilience. Scientific Support: Shilajit contains fulvic acid, which supports energy metabolism and may reduce stress-induced cortisol elevation.

Adrenal (55%) – Widely used for supporting adrenal hormone output and energy stability. Scientific Support: Adrenal extracts provide building blocks for adrenal hormone production and help buffer stress.

Tyrosine (28%) – Helps users stay mentally sharp and emotionally balanced under pressure. Scientific Support: Tyrosine supports dopamine and norepinephrine production, aiding focus and stress resilience.

Theanine (21%) – Commonly used to promote a relaxed, focused state without sedation. Scientific Support: Theanine increases alpha brain wave activity, supporting calm awareness.

Grounding Mat (15%) – Many users report greater calm and reduced body tension. Scientific Support: Grounding has been associated with reduced cortisol levels and improved mood balance.

Summary Table: Support Chronic Stress

Therapy	Solution	Details
Herbal Therapy	Ashwagandha	30% report reduced overwhelm; lowers cortisol and promotes calm.
Herbal Therapy	Licorice	24% report improved adrenal support; sustains cortisol regulation.

Therapy	Solution	Details
Herbal Therapy	Rhodiola	22% report more stamina; reduces stress-induced fatigue.
Mushroom Therapy	Reishi	20% report calmness and balance; supports nervous system regulation.
Amino Acid Therapy	GABA	20% report greater relaxation; helps reduce overstimulation.
HOPED Protocol	Shilajit	25% report improved resilience; supports energy and cortisol balance.
Animal Organ Therapy	Adrenal	55% report better tolerance to stress; supports adrenal hormone output.
Amino Acid Therapy	Tyrosine	28% report mental clarity; supports neurotransmitter balance.
Amino Acid Therapy	Theanine	21% report calm focus; promotes alpha brain wave activity.
Grounding Therapy	Grounding Mat	15% report lower tension and stress; associated with cortisol reduction.

To learn what research and real-world experience reveal about each of these solutions, and which one might be a good fit for you, see the corresponding therapy books in The Medicine-Free, Illness-Free Series.

Calmness and Emotional Resilience

Anxiety is often described as persistent worry, mental tension, and heightened sensitivity to stress. It may arise from imbalances in neurotransmitters such as GABA and serotonin, overactivity in the sympathetic nervous system, or chronic overstimulation of the brain's stress pathways.

Individuals experiencing anxiety frequently report symptoms such as racing thoughts, restlessness, difficulty relaxing, increased heart rate, and muscle tension. Natural therapies aim to calm the nervous system, support emotional regulation, and restore balance to the brain's chemical messengers, without the side effects associated with conventional medications.

Top Solutions for Emotional Calm and Resilience

Ashwagandha (25%) – Often used to support a calm and balanced mental state. Scientific Support: Clinical studies show Ashwagandha may help reduce symptoms of generalized anxiety by modulating cortisol and supporting neurotransmitter function.

Rhodiola (22%) – Known to ease emotional stress while preserving mental clarity. Scientific Support: Rhodiola may help regulate the body's stress response and support emotional resilience through effects on dopamine and serotonin pathways.

Reishi (20%) – Used to promote nervous system relaxation and inner calm. Scientific Support: Reishi interacts with GABA-related pathways to reduce overactivity and support emotional stability.

GABA (20%) – Frequently reported to promote a sense of calm and reduce overstimulation. Scientific Support: GABA is an inhibitory neurotransmitter that supports relaxation by reducing excitatory signaling.

Theanine (19%) – Helps promote a centered, calm state without drowsiness. Scientific Support: Theanine supports GABA and dopamine balance, contributing to a relaxed yet alert mental state.

Taurine (15%) – Supports emotional regulation and physical relaxation. Scientific Support: Taurine enhances GABA receptor sensitivity, helping ease stress-related nervous system activation.

Shilajit (25%) – Commonly used for mood stability and mental calm. Scientific Support: Shilajit contains trace minerals and fulvic acid that support neurotransmitter balance and adrenal regulation.

Grounding Mat (15%) – Users report reduced anxiety and physical tension. Scientific Support: Grounding has been linked to reduced sympathetic activity and may help ease psychological stress.

Summary Table: Calmness and Emotional Resilience

Therapy	Solution	Details
Herbal Therapy	Ashwagandha	25% of users report reduced anxiety; supports calm and cortisol balance.
Herbal Therapy	Rhodiola	22% of users report improved stress tolerance; modulates neurotransmitters.
Mushroom Therapy	Reishi	20% of users report emotional ease; supports GABA-related calming.
Amino Acid Therapy	GABA	20% of users report nervous system relief; promotes inhibitory signaling.
Amino Acid Therapy	Theanine	19% of users report calm focus; supports neurotransmitter balance.
Amino Acid Therapy	Taurine	15% of users report less tension; enhances GABA receptor activity.
HOPED Protocol	Shilajit	25% of users report mood support; helps regulate stress chemistry.
Grounding Therapy	Grounding Mat	15% of users report less anxiety; supports nervous system regulation.

To learn what research and real-world experience reveal about each of these solutions, and which one might be a good fit for you, see the corresponding therapy books in The Medicine-Free, Illness-Free Series.

Low Mood and Motivation

Low mood and reduced motivation are often associated with imbalances in neurotransmitters such as dopamine, serotonin, and norepinephrine. Chronic stress, fatigue, and systemic inflammation can also contribute to emotional flatness, decreased energy, and mental fog. Individuals experiencing low mood may report apathy, sleep disturbances, difficulty concentrating, and a general lack of drive.

Natural therapies that support emotional balance aim to enhance neurotransmitter production, improve energy metabolism, and help stabilize the body's stress response. These solutions are widely used to promote a brighter mood, improved motivation, and emotional clarity.

Top Solutions for Emotional Low Mood and Motivation

Phenylalanine (47%) – Often used to improve emotional stability and mental energy. Scientific Support: Phenylalanine is a precursor to tyrosine, which converts into dopamine and norepinephrine, neurotransmitters closely linked to mood and motivation.

Adrenal Extract (43%) – Reported to support emotional regulation and resilience, especially during adrenal fatigue. Scientific Support: Adrenal gland extracts contain cofactors that help support cortisol balance and stress hormone signaling, contributing to improved emotional recovery.

Tyrosine (28%) – Used to support motivation and mental performance under stress. Scientific Support: Tyrosine helps maintain dopamine production, which may aid emotional resilience and support mental clarity.

Shilajit (25%) – Frequently reported to reduce fatigue and support mood balance. Scientific Support: Shilajit provides trace minerals and fulvic acid that support energy metabolism and may influence mood-related pathways.

Tryptophan (19%) – Commonly taken to promote emotional comfort and well-being. Scientific Support: Tryptophan is a direct precursor to serotonin, a neurotransmitter that supports emotional regulation and positivity.

Summary Table: Low Mood and Motivation

Therapy	Solution	Details
Amino Acid Therapy	Phenylalanine	47% of users report improved mood; supports dopamine and neurotransmitter activity.
Animal Organ Therapy	Adrenal	43% of users report emotional stability; supports cortisol and stress resilience.
Amino Acid Therapy	Tyrosine	28% of users report better motivation; supports dopamine under stress.
HOPED Protocol	Shilajit	25% of users report more energy and clarity; supports mood and mitochondria.
Amino Acid Therapy	Tryptophan	19% of users report emotional balance; supports serotonin production.

To learn what research and real-world experience reveal about each of these solutions, and which one might be a good fit for you, see the corresponding therapy books in The Medicine-Free, Illness-Free Series.

Mood Stability and Irritability

Mood instability can stem from hormonal fluctuations, neurotransmitter imbalances, and chronic stress. Individuals experiencing mood swings may find it difficult to regulate their emotions, often struggling with irritability, impulsive reactions, and emotional volatility in response to everyday stressors. Anger and frustration, which often fall under this category, are frequently linked to low levels of GABA and serotonin, both important for maintaining emotional control and mental calm.

Natural therapies aimed at mood stabilization help by supporting neurotransmitter function, regulating cortisol and other stress-related hormones, and promoting balanced emotional responses over time.

Top Solutions for Mood Swings and Emotional Reactivity

Phenylalanine (47%) – Often used to support emotional regulation and consistent mood. Scientific Support: Phenylalanine is a precursor to tyrosine, which supports the synthesis of mood-related neurotransmitters including dopamine and serotonin.

Ashwagandha (32%) – Commonly used to ease irritability and emotional tension. Scientific Support: Ashwagandha supports cortisol regulation and has been shown to improve mood stability under stress.

Maca (14%) – Reported to promote mood consistency, especially during hormonal changes. Scientific Support: Maca nourishes the endocrine system and has demonstrated effects on mood swings, particularly in perimenopausal women.

Female Organs (23%) – Frequently used to support emotional balance in hormonally sensitive individuals. Scientific Support: Female organ extracts supply cofactors and nutrients that support estrogen and progesterone balance, helping reduce mood fluctuations.

Tryptophan (19%) – Taken to reduce emotional volatility and improve mood steadiness. Scientific Support: Tryptophan is a direct precursor to serotonin, which plays a key role in mood regulation and emotional calm.

Theanine (21%) – Used to promote emotional clarity and a more even mood. Scientific Support: Theanine enhances alpha brain wave activity and supports neurotransmitter balance, contributing to a calm yet alert state.

Summary Table: Mood Stability and Irritability

Therapy	Solution	Details
Amino Acid Therapy	Phenylalanine	47% of users report improved mood regulation; supports dopamine and serotonin.
Herbal Therapy	Ashwagandha	32% of users report less irritability; balances cortisol and emotional tone.
Herbal Therapy	Maca	14% of users report fewer mood swings; supports hormonal and mood stability.

Therapy	Solution	Details
Animal Organ Therapy	Female Organs	23% of users report better emotional balance; supports estrogen and progesterone.
Amino Acid Therapy	Tryptophan	19% of users report improved calm; supports serotonin production.
Amino Acid Therapy	Theanine	21% of users report reduced mood fluctuations; promotes a relaxed focus.

To learn what research and real-world experience reveal about each of these solutions, and which one might be a good fit for you, see the corresponding therapy books in The Medicine-Free, Illness-Free Series.

Sleep and Restfulness

Sleep is a foundational aspect of health, supporting cognitive function, immune strength, emotional regulation, and physical restoration. Yet many individuals experience challenges such as insomnia, poor sleep quality, or disrupted rest, which can contribute to fatigue, mood imbalances, and increased health risks over time.

The body's internal sleep-wake cycle, known as the circadian rhythm, is influenced by melatonin, serotonin, cortisol, and neurotransmitters like GABA and glycine. Disruptions in these systems, often caused by stress, hormonal shifts, overstimulation, or environmental cues, can interfere with the body's ability to enter deep, restorative sleep.

While pharmaceutical sleep aids may offer temporary support, they are not always well tolerated and may lead to dependency. In contrast, natural therapies work in harmony with the body's own systems to promote calm, regulate circadian timing, and support deeper, more restful sleep without unwanted side effects.

Below are natural solutions commonly used to support sleep and restfulness. Each is backed by scientific research and real-world experiences, categorized by specific sleep challenges.

Difficulty Falling or Staying Asleep

Insomnia refers to difficulty falling asleep, staying asleep, or waking up too early without feeling refreshed. It often leads to chronic fatigue, reduced focus, mood changes, and elevated stress levels. Contributing factors may include elevated cortisol, low serotonin or melatonin, or an overactive nervous system that prevents the body from entering a restful state.

Natural solutions for insomnia aim to support relaxation, restore healthy sleep-wake signaling, and calm the brain's stress response. These approaches help the body shift into rest mode without reliance on sedatives or habit-forming substances.

Top Solutions for Sleep Challenges

Ashwagandha (8%) – Often used to reduce nighttime tension and improve sleep onset. Scientific support: Ashwagandha helps lower cortisol and supports a calmer nervous system, contributing to better overall sleep quality.

Reishi (35%) – Frequently used to encourage deeper, uninterrupted sleep. Scientific support: Reishi has been studied for its ability to improve sleep quality and reduce fatigue through calming effects on the nervous system.

Glycine (85%) – Widely reported to improve sleep depth and quality. Scientific support: Glycine helps lower core body temperature and quiet the nervous system, facilitating smoother sleep transitions.

Tryptophan (55%) – Commonly used to support sleep initiation. Scientific support: Tryptophan is a precursor to serotonin and melatonin, both of which play key roles in regulating the sleep cycle.

GABA (43%) – Used to calm nighttime mental activity and reduce awakenings. Scientific support: GABA is an inhibitory neurotransmitter that helps quiet neural excitability, promoting longer, deeper sleep.

Theanine (35%) – Taken to support mental relaxation before bed. Scientific support: Theanine promotes alpha brain wave activity and reduces psychological tension, supporting easier sleep onset.

Grounding Mat (42%) – Users often report better sleep quality and less nighttime restlessness. Scientific support: Grounding may help normalize cortisol rhythms and support deeper sleep through nervous system regulation.

Summary Table: Difficulty Falling or Staying Asleep

Therapy	Solution	Details
Herbal Therapy	Ashwagandha	8% of users report easier sleep onset; supports cortisol balance and nighttime calm.
Mushroom Therapy	Reishi	35% of users report deeper, more restorative sleep; supports nervous system relaxation.
Amino Acid Therapy	Glycine	85% of users report better sleep quality; calms the nervous system and lowers body temperature.
Amino Acid Therapy	Tryptophan	55% of users report better sleep initiation; supports serotonin and melatonin production.
Amino Acid Therapy	GABA	43% of users report improved sleep continuity; reduces neural overactivity.
Amino Acid Therapy	Theanine	35% of users report better sleep quality; enhances relaxation and alpha brain activity.
Grounding Therapy	Grounding Mat	42% of users report better sleep patterns; supports circadian rhythm balance.

To learn what research and real-world experience reveal about each of these solutions, and which one might be a good fit for you, see the corresponding therapy books in The Medicine-Free, Illness-Free Series.

Poor Sleep Quality

Poor sleep quality occurs when someone gets an adequate number of hours but still wakes up feeling tired, foggy, or unrefreshed. This is often due to shallow sleep, frequent micro-awakenings, neurotransmitter imbalances, or disrupted melatonin production that prevents the body from reaching deeper restorative stages of rest.

Natural therapies that support sleep quality work by calming the nervous system, improving sleep architecture, and promoting uninterrupted, restful cycles. These approaches help restore the body's ability to enter and maintain the deep stages of sleep needed for full recovery.

Top Solutions for Poor Sleep Quality

Ashwagandha (20%) – Commonly used to reduce stress-related sleep disturbances. Scientific support: Ashwagandha supports cortisol regulation and nervous system balance, helping promote deeper, more restful sleep.

Moringa (14%) – Reported to enhance overall sleep depth. Scientific support: Moringa is a source of tryptophan and magnesium, which support serotonin production and healthy circadian rhythms.

Reishi (35%) – Frequently used to support restorative sleep and reduce nighttime wakefulness. Scientific support: Reishi's adaptogenic properties have been shown to improve sleep quality and support nervous system regulation.

Chaga (15%) – Used to promote a more balanced sleep-wake rhythm. Scientific support: Chaga's antioxidant properties may help reduce inflammation and oxidative stress that interfere with sleep.

Adrenal Extract (10%) – Often used to improve sleep patterns linked to stress. Scientific support: Adrenal extracts support cortisol rhythm regulation, which is critical for healthy sleep cycles.

Thyroid Extract (10%) – Beneficial for individuals whose sleep is affected by thyroid-related imbalances. Scientific support: Healthy thyroid function is associated with improved energy balance and sleep restoration.

Glycine (85%) – Widely used to enhance sleep depth and nighttime relaxation. Scientific support: Glycine lowers core body temperature and calms the nervous system, encouraging deeper sleep.

Serine (41%) – Reported to help the body transition smoothly into sleep. Scientific support: Serine supports neurotransmitter function involved in regulating sleep-wake cycles.

Taurine (28%) – Taken to ease nighttime tension and promote better quality sleep. Scientific support: Taurine modulates GABA activity and supports nervous system relaxation.

Summary Table: Poor Sleep Quality

Therapy	Solution	Details
Herbal Therapy	Ashwagandha	20% of users report more restful sleep; supports cortisol and calm.

Therapy	Solution	Details
Herbal Therapy	Moringa	14% of users report better sleep depth; supports serotonin balance.
Mushroom Therapy	Reishi	35% of users report improved sleep quality; supports nervous system recovery.
Mushroom Therapy	Chaga	15% of users report more refreshing sleep; supports antioxidant activity.
Animal Organ Therapy	Adrenal	10% of users report more consistent rest; supports cortisol regulation.
Animal Organ Therapy	Thyroid	10% of users report improved rest when thyroid function is balanced.
Amino Acid Therapy	Glycine	85% of users report deep relaxation; helps lower body temperature and ease sleep.
Amino Acid Therapy	Serine	41% of users report easier sleep transitions; supports neurotransmitter balance.
Amino Acid Therapy	Taurine	28% of users report better sleep quality; supports GABA receptor activity.

To learn what research and real-world experience reveal about each of these solutions, and which one might be a good fit for you, see the corresponding therapy books in The Medicine-Free, Illness-Free Series.

Restless Sleep and Nighttime Disruption

Restless sleep is often marked by frequent tossing and turning, shallow sleep cycles, and difficulty remaining in deeper, restorative stages of rest. This type of disruption is commonly associated with elevated nighttime cortisol, hormonal imbalances, or a nervous system that remains overstimulated during sleep.

Natural therapies that address these issues aim to calm the body's stress response, regulate hormonal rhythms, and support consistent, uninterrupted sleep throughout the night.

Top Solutions for Restless Sleep

Taurine (28%) – Frequently used to promote nighttime calm and reduce sleep disruptions. Scientific support: Taurine supports GABA receptor activity and helps regulate nervous system balance, promoting deeper relaxation during sleep.

Adrenal Extract (10%) – Used to balance cortisol rhythms and prevent overstimulation at night. Scientific support: Adrenal extracts provide cofactors that help regulate stress hormone cycles, supporting steadier sleep patterns.

Thyroid Extract (10%) – Often used by individuals whose restless sleep may be linked to thyroid imbalance. Scientific support: Balanced thyroid function supports natural energy rhythms and contributes to better nighttime recovery.

Shilajit (13%) – Commonly taken to ease nighttime stress and improve cortisol balance. Scientific support: Shilajit's trace minerals and fulvic acid help regulate stress hormones, contributing to more consistent rest.

Grounding Therapy (42%) – Widely reported to improve sleep continuity and reduce nighttime movement. Scientific support: Grounding has been shown to help align circadian rhythms, reduce cortisol spikes, and support parasympathetic nervous system activation.

Summary Table: Restless Sleep

Therapy	Solution	Details
Amino Acid Therapy	Taurine	28% of users report reduced restlessness; supports GABA activity and calm.
Animal Organ Therapy	Adrenal Extract	10% of users report improved sleep continuity; supports cortisol balance.
Animal Organ Therapy	Thyroid Extract	10% of users report deeper rest; supports thyroid regulation for sleep.
HOPED Protocol	Shilajit	13% of users report more restful nights; modulates nighttime stress hormones.
Grounding Therapy	Grounding Mat	42% of users report reduced nighttime restlessness; supports circadian alignment.

To learn what research and real-world experience reveal about each of these solutions, and which one might be a good fit for you, see the corresponding therapy books in The Medicine-Free, Illness-Free Series.

Inflammation and Structural Support

Inflammation is the body's natural defense mechanism in response to injury, infection, or imbalance. However, when inflammation becomes chronic or excessive, it can contribute to ongoing pain, swelling, stiffness, and eventual tissue damage. This persistent inflammatory state is associated with conditions such as arthritis, autoimmune disorders, and musculoskeletal imbalances, often resulting in reduced mobility and lower quality of life.

Pain associated with inflammation may take many forms, including chronic discomfort, joint pain, and systemic inflammatory conditions like rheumatoid arthritis or other autoimmune syndromes. While conventional options such as NSAIDs and corticosteroids are widely used, they may not address the underlying imbalance and often come with long-term side effects.

Natural therapies provide alternative approaches that are non-toxic, research-informed, and supportive of the body's innate healing response. These solutions work to reduce inflammation, ease discomfort, support joint function, and promote greater physical resilience.

Below are science-informed and user-validated natural solutions, organized by specific inflammation-related concerns.

Chronic Discomfort and Inflammatory Burden

Chronic pain is pain that persists beyond the expected period of healing, often lasting for weeks, months, or even years. It may result from nerve dysfunction, systemic inflammation, or unresolved musculoskeletal issues. Unlike acute pain, which serves as an immediate signal of injury, chronic pain tends to be ongoing and can significantly affect physical functioning, energy levels, and emotional well-being.

Natural therapies that address chronic discomfort focus on calming systemic inflammation, supporting detoxification, and improving circulation to reduce the buildup of pain-inducing compounds in the body. These approaches aim to support long-term comfort while minimizing the need for medications that may carry side effects.

Top Solutions for Chronic Discomfort

Turmeric (25%) – Used to ease ongoing pain and inflammation. Scientific support: Curcumin, the active compound in turmeric, is known to inhibit NF-kB and other inflammatory mediators associated with chronic pain.

Lymphatic Detox (16%) – Taken to support the body's removal of inflammatory waste. Scientific support: A healthy lymphatic system helps clear byproducts that contribute to inflammation and persistent discomfort.

Kidney Detox (15%) – Often used to reduce fluid retention and discomfort related to inflammation. Scientific support: Kidney detoxification supports efficient waste elimination, which may help reduce pain-inducing inflammatory compounds.

Grounding Mat (8%) – Reported to improve comfort by supporting recovery and reducing inflammation. Scientific support: Grounding therapy has been associated with reductions in cortisol and inflammatory markers such as C-reactive protein (CRP).

Summary Table: Chronic Discomfort and Inflammation

Therapy	Solution	Details
Herbal Therapy	Turmeric	25% of users report pain relief; curcumin reduces systemic inflammation.
Detox Therapy	Lymphatic Detox	16% of users report reduced discomfort; supports removal of inflammatory waste.
Detox Therapy	Kidney Detox	15% of users report less swelling; enhances elimination of pain triggers.
Grounding Therapy	Grounding Mat	8% of users report improved comfort; reduces cortisol and inflammation.

To learn what research and real-world experience reveal about each of these solutions, and which one might be a good fit for you, see the corresponding therapy books in The Medicine-Free, Illness-Free Series.

Joint Discomfort and Mobility

Arthritis is a common inflammatory condition that causes joint pain, stiffness, and reduced range of motion. It occurs when the protective cartilage in the joints wears down or becomes inflamed. Osteoarthritis is typically age-related and results from mechanical wear, while rheumatoid arthritis involves immune system activity that targets joint tissues.

Natural therapies for arthritis and joint discomfort aim to reduce inflammation, improve joint flexibility, and support tissue recovery. These approaches work by addressing inflammatory mediators and providing nutrients that contribute to joint structure and resilience.

Top Solutions for Arthritis and Joint Pain

Turmeric (45%) – Widely used to ease joint pain and improve daily movement. Scientific support: Curcumin, the active compound in turmeric, has demonstrated anti-inflammatory effects comparable to NSAIDs in clinical studies and may reduce swelling and joint stiffness.

Moringa (24%) – Frequently used for joint stiffness and comfort. Scientific support: Moringa contains antioxidant and anti-inflammatory compounds that help relieve discomfort in individuals with joint conditions.

Fish Oil (Omega-3s) (9%) – Commonly taken to support flexibility and reduce joint tension. Scientific support: Omega-3 fatty acids help regulate inflammation by lowering cytokine activity, which may contribute to improved joint comfort in both osteoarthritis and rheumatoid arthritis.

Summary Table: Joint Discomfort and Mobility

Therapy	Solution	Details
Herbal Therapy	Turmeric	45% of users report pain reduction and better mobility; curcumin eases inflammation.
Herbal Therapy	Moringa	24% of users report less stiffness; bioactives reduce inflammatory signals.
HOPED Protocol	Fish Oil	9% of users report improved flexibility; Omega-3s reduce inflammatory cytokines.

To learn what research and real-world experience reveal about each of these solutions, and which one might be a good fit for you, see

the corresponding therapy books in The Medicine-Free, Illness-Free Series.

Immune-Related Inflammation

Chronic inflammatory conditions such as rheumatoid arthritis, lupus, and other autoimmune disorders occur when the immune system mistakenly targets the body's own tissues. This can lead to persistent inflammation, joint discomfort, fatigue, and tissue damage over time.

Natural therapies for immune-related inflammation aim to support immune balance, calm inflammatory signaling, and promote the elimination of waste and byproducts that may contribute to immune dysregulation. These strategies help reduce chronic symptoms while supporting long-term wellness.

Top Solutions for Immune-Related Inflammation

Turmeric (25%) – Commonly used to support immune balance and relieve chronic inflammation. Scientific support: Curcumin, the active compound in turmeric, helps inhibit inflammatory cytokines and pathways associated with autoimmune responses.

Lymphatic Detox (16%) – Frequently used to support immune regulation and reduce discomfort from systemic inflammation. Scientific support: A healthy lymphatic system aids in clearing metabolic waste and excess immune activity that may contribute to autoimmune symptoms.

Grounding Mat (8%) – Used to improve immune resilience and reduce inflammatory burden. Scientific support: Grounding has been associated with lower levels of pro-inflammatory markers and may support immune system balance and tissue healing.

Summary Table: Immune-related Inflammation

Therapy	Solution	Details
Herbal Therapy	Turmeric	25% of users report immune balance; curcumin reduces inflammatory signaling.
Detox Therapy	Lymphatic Detox	16% of users report relief; promotes waste clearance and immune regulation.
Grounding Therapy	Grounding Mat	8% of users report less inflammation; supports immune balance and tissue repair.

To learn what research and real-world experience reveal about each of these solutions, and which one might be a good fit for you, see the corresponding therapy books in The Medicine-Free, Illness-Free Series.

Cardiovascular Health

The cardiovascular system plays a vital role in delivering oxygen and nutrients to every cell in the body, maintaining blood pressure, and supporting overall metabolic function. It includes the heart, arteries, veins, and capillaries, all working together to sustain life and performance.

Modern factors such as chronic stress, poor nutrition, physical inactivity, and exposure to toxins can negatively impact cardiovascular health. These influences often contribute to high blood pressure, elevated cholesterol, poor circulation, and increased risk for serious events like heart attack or stroke.

While conventional medications such as antihypertensives and statins are widely used, they can come with side effects and long-term risks. Natural approaches offer supportive, non-toxic alternatives that promote heart function, enhance circulation, and help maintain lipid balance when used as part of a healthy lifestyle.

Below are science-informed and customer-validated natural solutions, organized by specific cardiovascular concerns.

Healthy Blood Pressure Support

Hypertension, or consistently elevated blood pressure, increases the risk of cardiovascular complications such as heart attack, stroke, and kidney dysfunction. Contributing factors often include impaired blood vessel function, excess sodium intake, chronic stress, and low nitric oxide production, which affects vascular relaxation.

Natural therapies for supporting healthy blood pressure focus on enhancing nitric oxide availability, improving vascular tone, and supporting overall cardiovascular resilience. These approaches may help maintain blood pressure within a healthy range without the side effects associated with conventional medication.

Top Solutions for Blood Pressure Support

Beet Root (35%) – Frequently used to support healthy blood pressure through nitric oxide production. Scientific support: Clinical studies show that beetroot nitrates improve endothelial function and help lower systolic and diastolic pressure.

Arginine (15%) – Often used to improve circulation and vascular function. Scientific support: Arginine is a key precursor to nitric oxide, which supports blood vessel dilation and blood pressure regulation.

Heart (12%) – Taken to support cardiac tone and overall heart health. Scientific support: Nutrients and peptides in heart tissue extracts may support blood pressure balance and heart muscle function.

CoQ10 (49%) – Popular for improving cardiovascular function and supporting blood pressure. Scientific support: CoQ10 enhances mitochondrial energy in cardiac cells and has been shown to reduce blood pressure in clinical studies.

Grounding Mat (5%) – Used to help support circulation and relaxation. Scientific support: Grounding has been associated with improved autonomic nervous system balance, which supports vascular relaxation and improved blood flow.

Summary Table: Blood Pressure Support

Therapy	Solution	Details
Herbal Therapy	Beet Root	35% of users report lower blood pressure; supports nitric oxide production.
Amino Acid Therapy	Arginine	15% of users report improved circulation; supports vascular tone.
Animal Organ Therapy	Heart	12% of users report cardiovascular support; nutrients support heart rhythm.
HOPED Protocol	CoQ10	49% of users report better heart function; supports mitochondrial energy and blood pressure.
Grounding Therapy	Grounding Mat	5% of users report improved circulation; supports nervous system balance.

To learn what research and real-world experience reveal about each of these solutions, and which one might be a good fit for you, see the corresponding therapy books in The Medicine-Free, Illness-Free Series.

Lipid Balance and Heart Function

Cholesterol is a necessary compound for hormone production, brain health, and cell membrane integrity. However, imbalances, such as elevated low-density lipoprotein (LDL) and reduced high-density lipoprotein (HDL), can lead to arterial plaque buildup and increased cardiovascular risk. Oxidized LDL, in particular, contributes to inflammation and narrowing of the arteries, a process known as atherosclerosis.

Natural therapies for lipid support focus on promoting healthy cholesterol ratios, reducing oxidative stress, and protecting vascular function. These approaches offer a supportive alternative for maintaining heart health alongside a balanced lifestyle.

Top Solutions for Lipid Balance

Resveratrol (28%) – Commonly used to support cholesterol balance and vascular function. Scientific support: Resveratrol has been shown to reduce oxidative stress, prevent LDL oxidation, and enhance endothelial function.

Fish Oil (16%) – Often used to help improve lipid profiles and support healthy arterial function. Scientific support: Omega-3 fatty acids in fish oil are associated with reductions in LDL, increases in HDL, and lower triglycerides.

Fish Eggs (10%) – Chosen for heart and vascular support due to high concentrations of omega-3s. Scientific support: Fish eggs provide bioavailable EPA and DHA, which support vascular flexibility and healthy lipid metabolism.

Summary Table: Lipid Balance and Heart Function Support

Therapy	Solution	Details
HOPED Protocol	Resveratrol	28% of users report improved cholesterol balance; reduces oxidative stress and supports vascular function.
HOPED Protocol	Fish Oil	16% of users report improved lipid profiles; lowers LDL and triglycerides, increases HDL.
HOPED Protocol	Fish Eggs	10% of users report enhanced heart function; delivers EPA and DHA to support healthy cholesterol and circulation.

To learn what research and real-world experience reveal about each of these solutions, and which one might be a good fit for you, see the corresponding therapy books in The Medicine-Free, Illness-Free Series.

Heart and Circulatory Support

Heart-related conditions such as coronary artery disease, heart failure, and irregular heartbeat affect the heart's ability to pump blood efficiently, impacting oxygen and nutrient delivery to the rest of the body. Contributing factors include oxidative stress, inflammation, poor circulation, and impaired mitochondrial function within cardiac tissue.

Natural therapies for cardiovascular support aim to strengthen heart muscle function, improve energy production, and enhance blood flow. These approaches help promote long-term cardiovascular resilience and support optimal circulation.

Top Solutions for Heart and Circulatory Support

CoQ10 (49%) – Commonly used to support heart energy and overall cardiovascular performance. Scientific support: CoQ10 plays a key role in mitochondrial ATP production and has been shown to improve heart function in individuals with cardiovascular challenges.

Beef Heart (57%) – Often chosen to support cardiac muscle tone and stamina. Scientific support: Heart organ extracts contain peptides and nutrients that may assist in oxygen delivery, endurance, and healthy circulation.

Beet Root (16%) – Used to support blood vessel flexibility and oxygenation. Scientific support: Beet root is rich in nitrates that convert to nitric oxide, supporting vasodilation and improving blood flow.

Arginine (11%) – Supports nitric oxide production and vascular function. Scientific support: Arginine has been studied for its role in enhancing endothelial function and maintaining vascular tone.

Summary Table: Heart and Circulatory Support

Therapy	Solution	Details
HOPED Protocol	CoQ10	49% of users report improved heart energy and function; supports ATP production.
Animal Organ Therapy	Heart	57% of users report better endurance and circulation; supports oxygen delivery.
Herbal Therapy	Beet Root	16% of users report improved blood flow; enhances nitric oxide for vasodilation.
Amino Acid Therapy	Arginine	11% of users report better cardiovascular performance; supports vascular health.

To learn what research and real-world experience reveal about each of these solutions, and which one might be a good fit for you, see the corresponding therapy books in The Medicine-Free, Illness-Free Series.

Skin, Hair, and Nail Health

The skin, hair, and nails reflect the body's internal health, influenced by nutrient intake, hormonal balance, detoxification efficiency, and inflammation levels. These external tissues regenerate constantly and require a steady supply of supportive nutrients, antioxidants, and structural proteins to maintain strength, clarity, and resilience.

While conventional treatments often rely on topical creams, serums, or shampoos, lasting improvement comes from within. Cellular repair, collagen production, and detoxification processes play a foundational role in supporting healthy skin tone, hair growth, and nail integrity.

Concerns such as blemishes, slow wound healing, dryness, premature aging, hair thinning, and brittle nails often signal deeper imbalances. Natural therapies address these concerns by delivering targeted nutrients, supporting hormonal and antioxidant pathways, and promoting structural repair.

Below are the most effective natural solutions for skin, hair, and nail wellness. Each has been selected based on scientific support and real-world validation from thousands of users.

Skin Repair and Recovery Support

Skin concerns such as acne, slow-healing wounds, ulcers, and irritation caused by viral outbreaks often involve inflammation, microbial imbalance, and reduced tissue regeneration. Whether facing blemishes, minor skin damage, or recurring skin irritation, effective support begins with enhancing collagen production, strengthening the skin barrier, and supporting the body's natural repair processes.

Top Solution for Skin Recovery and Clarity

Lysine (22%) – Supports skin clarity, wound healing, and resilience to external stressors. Scientific support: Lysine plays a role in collagen synthesis and has been shown in studies to aid skin recovery and promote healthy tissue repair. It also supports immune defense mechanisms involved in skin health.

Summary Table: Skin Repair & Recovery

Therapy	Solution	Details
Amino Acid Therapy	Lysine	22%; supports wound healing, promotes collagen formation, and aids skin clarity

To learn what research and real-world experience reveal about this solution, and whether it might be a good fit for you, see the corresponding therapy books in The Medicine-Free, Illness-Free Series.

Skin Radiance and Vitality

Visible signs of skin aging, such as fine lines, uneven tone, sagging, and dryness, are often driven by oxidative stress, declining collagen production, and chronic inflammation. Restoring youthful skin requires more than surface treatments. Internal support through targeted nutrients and regenerative compounds can enhance elasticity, brighten complexion, and support overall skin renewal.

Natural solutions for skin vitality focus on increasing collagen synthesis, protecting against oxidative damage, and nourishing the skin from within to promote lasting radiance and resilience.

Top Solutions for Skin Vitality and Hydration

Resveratrol (32%) – Reduces oxidative stress, supports collagen stability, and improves skin resilience. Scientific support: As a powerful antioxidant, resveratrol helps minimize fine lines, improve hydration, and protect skin from environmental damage.

Collagen (28%) – Improves hydration, firmness, and smoothness. Scientific support: Collagen peptides stimulate fibroblasts and enhance dermal density, contributing to visibly healthier, more radiant skin.

Glutathione (40%) – Brightens skin tone, reduces uneven pigmentation, and supports skin clarity. Scientific support: Known as the body's master antioxidant, glutathione regulates melanin production and neutralizes oxidative stress affecting skin appearance.

Bone & Marrow (24%) – Enhances skin hydration, elasticity, and texture. Scientific support: Bone and marrow extracts contain collagen-building blocks and minerals that support skin structure and regeneration.

Summary Table: Skin Vitality and Hydration

Therapy	Solution	Details
HOPED Protocol	Resveratrol	32%; reduces oxidative stress, improves skin resilience
Animal Organ Therapy	Collagen	28%; supports hydration, firmness, and radiance

Therapy	Solution	Details
Amino Acid Therapy	Glutathione	40%; brightens complexion, supports skin clarity
Animal Organ Therapy	Bone & Marrow	24%; enhances elasticity, hydration, and skin tone

To learn what research and real-world experience reveal about each of these solutions, and which one might be a good fit for you, see the corresponding therapy books in The Medicine-Free, Illness-Free Series.

Hair Health

Hair thinning, shedding, and slowed growth are commonly linked to hormonal shifts, nutrient deficiencies, oxidative stress, and poor circulation to hair follicles. One key factor in both male and female pattern hair changes is DHT (dihydrotestosterone), a hormone derived from testosterone that can shrink hair follicles over time.

Natural solutions for hair vitality aim to block DHT, restore essential nutrients, and improve follicle health from the inside out. These approaches support stronger, thicker, shinier hair while promoting regrowth and reducing breakage.

Top Solutions for Hair Vitality and Strength

Saw Palmetto (29%) – Blocks DHT and reduces shedding by inhibiting 5-alpha reductase, the enzyme that converts testosterone into DHT. Scientific support: Studies show Saw Palmetto supports hair density and slows androgen-related hair loss in both men and women.

Collagen (24%) – Supports fullness, strength, and shine while reducing breakage and thinning. Scientific support: Collagen provides the amino acids needed for keratin production and strengthens the hair shaft and follicle structure.

Liver (21%) – Improves hair density and appearance through nutrient repletion. Scientific support: Liver is naturally rich in biotin, vitamin A, iron, and other cofactors vital for follicle integrity and scalp circulation.

Organ Complex (12%) – Promotes overall follicle health with a spectrum of supportive organ-based nutrients. Scientific support: Multi-organ supplements offer a broad nutrient matrix that nourishes the entire hair growth system.

Summary Table: Hair Health

Therapy	Solution	Details
Herbal Therapy	Saw Palmetto	29%; blocks DHT, reduces shedding and supports regrowth
Animal Organ Therapy	Collagen	24%; improves shine, reduces breakage, supports hair thickness
Animal Organ Therapy	Liver	21%; rich in biotin and iron, strengthens follicles
Animal Organ Therapy	Organ Complex	12%; multi-organ support for follicle and scalp nourishment

To learn what research and real-world experience reveal about each of these solutions, and which one might be a good fit for you, see the corresponding therapy books in The Medicine-Free, Illness-Free Series.

Nail Health

Brittle, weak, or slow-growing nails often reflect underlying nutrient deficiencies, protein metabolism issues, or low-grade systemic inflammation. Strengthening nail structure from within requires support for keratin production, collagen synthesis, and optimal mineral balance.

Natural therapies for nail resilience focus on delivering bioavailable nutrients that promote durability, reduce breakage, and enhance overall appearance. When supported properly, nails become stronger, smoother, and less prone to splitting or peeling.

Top Solutions for Nail Strength and Growth

Collagen (17%) – Strengthens brittle nails and promotes faster, healthier growth. Scientific support: Collagen peptides enhance nail thickness and durability, stimulate keratin production, and reduce breakage according to clinical studies.

Liver (15%) – Improves nail strength and reduces brittleness by supplying biotin, iron, and essential cofactors for keratin formation. Scientific support: Liver is rich in micronutrients required for healthy nail matrix development and resilience.

Summary Table: Nail Health

Therapy	Solution	Details
Animal Organ Therapy	Collagen	17%; strengthens brittle nails and promotes faster, healthier growth
Animal Organ Therapy	Liver	15%; supports nail strength and prevents brittleness with biotin and iron

To learn what research and real-world experience reveal about each of these solutions, and which one might be a good fit for you, see the corresponding therapy books in The Medicine-Free, Illness-Free Series.

Oral, Dental and Upper Respiratory Support

Oral health is about more than having clean teeth. It plays a vital role in digestion, immune function, and even cardiovascular wellness. The mouth hosts a diverse microbiome, and when this delicate balance of bacteria is disrupted, it can lead to cavities, gum disease, bad breath, and systemic inflammation that extends beyond the oral cavity.

Traditional oral care routines, such as brushing, flossing, and using antibacterial mouthwash, are important, but they do not address the root causes of microbial imbalance. Disrupting beneficial bacteria may create short-term cleanliness at the expense of long-term oral resilience.

Research increasingly supports the role of oral probiotics and targeted natural therapies in maintaining a healthy oral environment. These solutions help balance microbial populations, reduce harmful plaque buildup, support gum integrity, and improve breath freshness. A healthy oral microbiome contributes to stronger immunity, healthier digestion, and reduced inflammation throughout the body.

Overall Oral Health

A balanced oral microbiome plays a vital role in preventing cavities, supporting enamel strength, reducing plaque buildup, and maintaining gum health. Harmful bacteria such as *Streptococcus mutans* contribute to tooth decay, while others associated with gingivitis can lead to gum inflammation and bleeding.

Natural therapies like oral probiotics work to restore microbial balance, helping reduce these risks while promoting a healthier mouth.

Top Solution for Overall Oral Health

Oral Probiotics (33%) – Improve oral health by restoring balance to the mouth's microbiome, helping to prevent plaque buildup, cavities, and gum disease. Scientific support: Clinical studies show that specific probiotic strains can colonize the oral cavity, reduce harmful bacteria, and promote healthier gums and fresher breath.

Summary Table: Oral Microbiome and Cavity Support

Therapy	Solution	Details
HOPED Protocol	Oral Probiotics	33%; fewer cavities, healthier gums, fresher breath

To learn what research and real-world experience reveal about this solution, and whether it might be a good fit for you, see the corresponding therapy books in The Medicine-Free, Illness-Free Series.

Gum Health & Comfort

Gum health is essential for preserving your teeth and supporting whole-body wellness. Inflammation of the gums, often caused by an imbalance of oral bacteria, can result in redness, swelling, bleeding, and gum recession. Over time, if left unaddressed, it may contribute to bone loss and more serious oral concerns.

Natural solutions focus on supporting a healthy oral microbiome and reducing inflammation without disrupting the natural bacterial balance in the mouth. These approaches promote long-term gum resilience and comfort.

Top Solution for Gum Health

Oral Probiotics (20%) – Help reduce gum inflammation, bleeding, and harmful bacterial overgrowth by supporting a balanced oral microbiome. Scientific support: Beneficial strains found in oral probiotics have been shown to inhibit the growth of bacteria linked to gingivitis, promoting healthier gums without disrupting natural microbial balance.

Summary Table: Gum Health and Comfort

Therapy	Solution	Details
HOPED Protocol	Oral Probiotics	20%; reduces gum inflammation and bleeding

To learn what research and real-world experience reveal about this solution, and whether it might be a good fit for you, see the corresponding therapy books in The Medicine-Free, Illness-Free Series.

Enamel Strength and Oral Cleanliness

Cavities occur when harmful bacteria break down sugars into acids, which erode tooth enamel and lead to decay. While fluoride and regular dental cleanings are commonly used for prevention, probiotic therapy offers a natural, targeted approach to reduce cavity-causing bacteria and support long-term oral health.

Top Solution for Cavity Prevention

Oral Probiotics (12%) – Help reduce plaque buildup and cavity risk by targeting harmful bacteria like *Streptococcus mutans*, which is responsible for tooth decay. Scientific support: Studies show that specific probiotic strains can inhibit cavity-causing bacteria, promoting a healthier oral environment and reducing the need for frequent dental interventions.

Summary Table: Enamel Strength and Oral Cleanliness

Therapy	Solution	Details
HOPED Protocol	Oral Probiotics	12%; lowers plaque and cavity risk

To learn what research and real-world experience reveal about this solution, and whether it might be a good fit for you, see the corresponding therapy books in The Medicine-Free, Illness-Free Series.

Fresh Breath and Oral Hygiene

Bad breath is often caused by odor-producing bacteria that break down food particles and proteins in the mouth. Conventional mouthwashes typically use alcohol-based antibacterial agents, but these can disrupt the oral microbiome and contribute to dry mouth, which may worsen halitosis over time.

Top Solution for Bad Breath Reduction

Oral Probiotics (27%) – Help eliminate bad breath by reducing odor-causing bacteria in the mouth. By promoting a balanced oral microbiome, probiotics lower levels of volatile sulfur compounds (VSCs), which are the main contributors to unpleasant breath. Scientific support: Research shows that certain probiotic strains can significantly reduce oral malodor by suppressing harmful bacteria and enhancing beneficial microbial activity.

Summary Table: Fresh Breath and Oral Hygiene

Therapy	Solution	Details
HOPED Protocol	Oral Probiotics	27%; reduces odor-causing bacteria for fresher breath

To learn what research and real-world experience reveal about this solution, and whether it might be a good fit for you, see the corresponding therapy books in The Medicine-Free, Illness-Free Series.

Throat & Sinus Support

Oral probiotics can colonize the nasopharyngeal region, helping to maintain a balanced microbiome that competes with harmful bacteria contributing to sinus congestion and throat irritation.

Top Solution for Throat & Sinus Health

Oral Probiotics (7%) – Support throat and sinus health by populating the nasopharyngeal region with beneficial bacteria that outcompete pathogens responsible for sore throats and sinus infections. Scientific support: Clinical studies suggest that oral probiotic strains can reduce the frequency and severity of upper respiratory tract infections by balancing the local microbiome.

Summary Table: Throat & Sinus Support

Therapy	Solution	Details
HOPED Protocol	Oral Probiotics	7%; eases throat irritation and sinus issues

To learn what research and real-world experience reveal about this solution, and whether it might be a good fit for you, see the corresponding therapy books in The Medicine-Free, Illness-Free Series.

Energy and Vitality

Energy is the foundation of health, vitality, and overall well-being. It fuels every function in the body, from mental clarity and immune resilience to muscle strength and cardiovascular performance. Yet, many people struggle with chronic fatigue, daily sluggishness, and low endurance, limiting their ability to function and enjoy life.

Unlike occasional tiredness, persistent low energy often points to deeper imbalances such as mitochondrial dysfunction, adrenal depletion, nutrient deficiencies, slow metabolism, or poor circulation. While caffeine and stimulants may provide quick boosts, they often result in crashes and long-term dependence without addressing the root cause.

Lasting energy requires support at the cellular level. This includes enhancing ATP production, improving oxygen utilization, optimizing nutrient absorption, and regulating metabolic function. Natural therapies can help rebuild energy from the inside out by supporting these key systems.

This section explores three common patterns of energy imbalance: chronic fatigue, low daily energy, and reduced physical endurance. Chronic fatigue refers to ongoing exhaustion that does not improve with rest and is often linked to adrenal or mitochondrial dysfunction. Low energy describes everyday sluggishness, brain fog, or afternoon crashes, frequently caused by circulation issues or nutrient depletion. Physical endurance, the ability to sustain activity over time, requires efficient ATP production and muscular resilience. The solutions in this section are backed by science and customer-reported results, offering a natural path to restoring energy and vitality.

Persistent Fatigue and Energy Recovery

Chronic fatigue is a persistent state of exhaustion that does not improve with rest and often leads to brain fog, physical weakness, and prolonged recovery from exertion. It is commonly linked to adrenal burnout, mitochondrial dysfunction, sluggish metabolism, and anemia. Addressing these root causes supports sustainable energy production, hormone balance, and cellular vitality without reliance on stimulants.

Top Solutions for Chronic Fatigue

Ginseng (40%) – Boosts vitality and stress resilience, reducing overall exhaustion. Scientific support: Helps regulate cortisol levels and supports ATP production, providing a natural energy lift.

Rhodiola (32%) – Enhances stamina and prevents energy crashes by supporting stress adaptation. Scientific support: Improves oxygen efficiency and mitochondrial function, contributing to long-lasting energy.

Cordyceps (40%) – Increases ATP production and oxygen utilization, especially beneficial for post-exertion recovery. Scientific support: Supports mitochondrial energy output and physical endurance.

Female Organs (60%) – Alleviates fatigue related to hormone fluctuations and menstrual cycles. Scientific support: Supplies hormone precursors that support stable energy and endocrine function.

Testicles (56%) – Supports male energy, endurance, and vitality by boosting testosterone. Scientific support: Provides androgens that enhance stamina and physical performance.

Liver (36%) – Combats sluggishness, especially in cases of low iron or anemia. Scientific support: Rich in bioavailable iron, B12, and coenzymes vital for cellular energy.

Brain (35%) – Improves mental clarity and physical alertness. Scientific support: Supports neurotransmitter synthesis to reduce fatigue and brain fog.

Thyroid (28%) – Regulates metabolism and energy production. Scientific support: Delivers cofactors that assist thyroid hormone synthesis and energy stability.

Spleen (27%) – Stabilizes daily energy and reduces fatigue by supporting blood health. Scientific support: Enhances red blood cell production for better oxygen delivery.

Adrenal (35%) – Restores balanced energy by supporting adrenal hormone production. Scientific support: Helps prevent adrenal fatigue and maintains steady cortisol output.

Arginine (39%) – Improves circulation and nutrient delivery, enhancing physical energy. Scientific support: Increases nitric oxide, improving blood flow and tissue oxygenation.

Tyrosine (29%) – Supports neurotransmitter balance for mental energy and focus. Scientific support: Precursor to dopamine and norepinephrine, essential for alertness and stamina.

Phenylalanine (27%) – Enhances mood and motivation, combating mental and physical fatigue. Scientific support: Involved in the production of dopamine and other energizing neurotransmitters.

Shilajit (44%) – Boosts energy at the cellular level by improving mitochondrial efficiency. Scientific support: Rich in fulvic acid, it enhances ATP production and nutrient absorption.

Summary Table: Chronic Fatigue

Therapy	Solution	Details
Herbal Therapy	Ginseng	40%; boosts daily vitality and stress resilience
Herbal Therapy	Rhodiola	32%; increases stamina and reduces energy crashes
Mushroom Therapy	Cordyceps	40%; enhances ATP production and oxygen transport
Animal Organ Therapy	Female Organs	60%; supports hormonal energy balance
Animal Organ Therapy	Testicles	56%; improves stamina and endurance
Animal Organ Therapy	Liver	36%; combats sluggishness and anemia-related fatigue
Animal Organ Therapy	Brain	35%; sharpens mental and physical energy
Animal Organ Therapy	Thyroid	28%; enhances metabolic function for sustained energy
Animal Organ Therapy	Spleen	27%; stabilizes energy levels and prevents anemia-related fatigue
Animal Organ Therapy	Adrenal	35%; combats chronic tiredness and adrenal burnout
Amino Acid Therapy	Arginine	39%; improves circulation and nutrient delivery for better energy
Amino Acid Therapy	Tyrosine	29%; enhances mental alertness and neurotransmitter balance
Amino Acid Therapy	Phenylalanine	27%; supports cognitive and physical energy levels
HOPED Protocol	Shilajit	44%; boosts mitochondrial function and stamina

To learn what research and real-world experience reveal about each of these solutions, and which one might be a good fit for you, see the corresponding therapy books in The Medicine-Free, Illness-Free Series.

Daily Energy and Stamina

Low energy levels are characterized by sluggishness, difficulty staying alert, and mid-day energy crashes. Unlike chronic fatigue, which persists for extended periods, low energy levels fluctuate throughout the day and often result from poor circulation, sluggish metabolism, mitochondrial inefficiency, and nutrient deficiencies.

The solutions for chronic fatigue also help improve low energy levels by enhancing ATP production, stabilizing metabolism, and supporting hormone balance. However, additional therapies specifically target nutrient absorption, oxygen efficiency, and cellular resilience, ensuring sustained daily energy without reliance on stimulants.

Top Solutions for Low Energy Levels

Spirulina (35%) – Provides a sustained energy boost through its rich blend of vitamins, minerals, and antioxidants that fuel cellular energy. Scientific support: Spirulina enhances mitochondrial function and supports ATP production, improving overall vitality.

Moringa (33%) – Boosts stamina and daily energy by replenishing essential micronutrients. Scientific support: Moringa is high in vitamins, minerals, and amino acids that combat fatigue and promote steady energy.

Beet Root (29%) – Improves oxygen transport and circulation, enhancing endurance and vitality. Scientific support: Nitrate content in beetroot promotes nitric oxide production, increasing oxygen utilization.

Organ Complex (53%) – Delivers a broad spectrum of nutrients that support mitochondrial function and steady energy output. Scientific support: Combines liver, heart, kidney, and other organ extracts to promote stamina and reduce fatigue.

Bone & Marrow (37%) – Supports endurance and physical recovery by providing structural and metabolic support. Scientific support: Contains collagen, minerals, and cofactors that enhance muscular energy and resilience.

Thymus (32%) – Promotes stable energy by supporting immune system balance and endocrine function. Scientific support: Thymic peptides help regulate metabolism and vitality.

Colostrum (25%) – Enhances energy and resilience through immune and tissue repair support. Scientific support: Contains growth factors and immunoglobulins that aid in cellular repair and energy metabolism.

Kidney (16%) – Helps balance fluid and adrenal health to reduce afternoon crashes. Scientific support: Provides bioavailable minerals that stabilize energy and support stress response.

Carnitine (54%) – Increases endurance by enhancing fat metabolism and ATP generation. Scientific support: Transports fatty acids into mitochondria for energy production.

D-Aspartic Acid (DAA) (33%) – Supports energy and stamina by promoting testosterone production. Scientific support: Influences hormonal pathways tied to metabolism and physical performance.

Taurine (28%) – Regulates cellular hydration and mitochondrial activity, helping reduce fatigue. Scientific support: Modulates calcium signaling and supports steady energy output.

Glutathione (22%) – Boosts energy by protecting mitochondria from oxidative damage. Scientific support: Acts as a master antioxidant that sustains metabolic efficiency.

Glutamine (17%) – Maintains energy during recovery by supporting muscles and digestion. Scientific support: Prevents muscle breakdown and supports gut health, aiding overall energy levels.

CoQ10 (35%) – Improves energy output by supporting heart function and mitochondrial ATP synthesis. Scientific support: Vital for cellular respiration and cardiovascular endurance.

Resveratrol (30%) – Enhances metabolic function and cellular energy, improving endurance. Scientific support: Supports mitochondrial health and reduces oxidative stress.

Vitamin D (20%) – Promotes steady energy by regulating hormones and immune function. Scientific support: Plays a key role in energy metabolism and mood stability.

Summary Table: Low Energy Levels

Therapy	Solution	Details
Herbal Therapy	Spirulina	35%; provides nutrient-dense energy support
Herbal Therapy	Moringa	33%; replenishes key vitamins and minerals
Herbal Therapy	Beet Root	29%; improves oxygen utilization and endurance

Therapy	Solution	Details
Animal Organ Therapy	Organ Complex	53%; comprehensive nutrient boost for steady energy
Animal Organ Therapy	Bone & Marrow	37%; enhances endurance and muscle recovery
Animal Organ Therapy	Thymus	32%; supports immune balance and sustained energy
Animal Organ Therapy	Colostrum	25%; improves vibrancy and reduces sluggishness
Animal Organ Therapy	Kidney	16%; stabilizes energy and prevents afternoon crashes
Amino Acid Therapy	Carnitine	54%; enhances fat metabolism for ATP production
Amino Acid Therapy	DAA	33%; boosts stamina via hormone modulation
Amino Acid Therapy	Taurine	28%; regulates cellular energy and fatigue
Amino Acid Therapy	Glutathione	22%; reduces oxidative stress and supports mitochondria
Amino Acid Therapy	Glutamine	17%; maintains energy levels via muscle and gut support
HOPED Protocol	CoQ10	35%; improves ATP synthesis and cardiovascular endurance
HOPED Protocol	Resveratrol	30%; boosts mitochondrial function and metabolic efficiency
HOPED Protocol	Vitamin D	20%; supports hormone regulation and sustained energy

To learn what research and real-world experience reveal about each of these solutions, and which one might be a good fit for you, see

the corresponding therapy books in The Medicine-Free, Illness-Free Series.

Physical Performance and Endurance

Physical endurance refers to the body's ability to sustain prolonged activity without experiencing excessive fatigue. It is essential for athletes, active individuals, and those seeking to improve daily stamina. Endurance is influenced by muscle recovery, oxygen utilization, cardiovascular efficiency, and energy metabolism. Supporting these factors naturally can enhance performance, delay fatigue, and improve overall physical resilience.

Top Solutions for Physical Endurance

EAAs (Essential Amino Acids) (35%) – Boost stamina and energy sustainability during extended physical activity by supporting muscle protein synthesis and overall metabolic performance. Scientific support: EAAs supply all nine essential amino acids required for muscle repair, ATP generation, and sustained energy output.

BCAAs (Branched-Chain Amino Acids) (56%) – Prevent muscle breakdown and delay fatigue during workouts, allowing for longer exercise duration and quicker recovery. Scientific support: BCAAs reduce exercise-induced muscle damage and central fatigue by preserving muscle tissue and improving endurance.

Heart (23%) – Enhances cardiovascular endurance and supports oxygen-rich blood flow during physical activity. Scientific support: Heart tissue is naturally high in CoQ10 and essential nutrients that improve mitochondrial function and cardiovascular efficiency, supporting sustained performance.

Summary Table: Physical Performance and Endurance

Therapy	Solution	Details
Amino Acid Therapy	EAAs	35%; boosts stamina and sustains energy
Amino Acid Therapy	BCAAs	56%; prevents muscle breakdown and delays fatigue
Animal Organ Therapy	Heart	23%; improves endurance and circulation

To learn what research and real-world experience reveal about each of these solutions, and which one might be a good fit for you, see the corresponding therapy books in The Medicine-Free, Illness-Free Series.

Respiratory Health

The respiratory system is essential for oxygen exchange, immune defense, and overall vitality. However, exposure to modern environmental factors, including pollutants, allergens, microbes, and indoor toxins, can impair lung function and respiratory efficiency. Conditions such as asthma, seasonal allergies, and chronic sinus issues often stem from inflammation, immune hypersensitivity, and mucus overproduction, making breathing more difficult and reducing quality of life.

While conventional treatments like bronchodilators, antihistamines, and corticosteroids can offer temporary symptom relief, they may not address the underlying imbalances and can lead to unwanted side effects with long-term use.

Natural therapies offer a gentler, holistic approach by helping to reduce inflammation, enhance lung capacity, support immune modulation, and protect delicate respiratory tissues. These therapies work with the body's natural healing processes to improve oxygen uptake, maintain airway clarity, and promote long-term respiratory wellness.

Breathing and Lung Support

Asthma is a chronic inflammatory condition of the lungs that causes airway narrowing, shortness of breath, wheezing, and persistent coughing. It is often triggered by allergens, infections, stress, or physical exertion. Inflammation in the airways leads to excess mucus and bronchial muscle constriction, making it difficult to breathe comfortably. While conventional treatments often rely on bronchodilators and corticosteroids, natural therapies can also support respiratory health by reducing inflammation, improving oxygen utilization, and strengthening lung tissue.

Top Solutions for Asthma

Cordyceps (15%) – Enhances oxygen utilization and supports respiratory function, making breathing easier for individuals with asthma. Scientific support: Cordyceps has been shown to improve lung efficiency by increasing oxygen uptake and reducing airway inflammation.

Agarikon (20%) – Expands lung capacity and eases persistent coughing, improving overall breathing comfort. Scientific support: Agarikon possesses anti-inflammatory and antimicrobial properties that help protect lung tissue and support respiratory resilience.

Lung (29%) – Strengthens respiratory function and promotes better airflow by nourishing lung tissue. Scientific support: Lung glandular supplements provide essential nutrients that support oxygen exchange, reduce inflammation, and improve overall lung health.

NAC (N-acetylcysteine) (21%) – Breaks down thick mucus in the lungs, improving airflow and breathing ease. Scientific support: NAC is a well-established mucolytic agent used clinically to thin mucus and enhance lung function in chronic respiratory conditions.

Summary Table: Breathing and Lung Support

Therapy	Solution	Details
Mushroom Therapy	Cordyceps	15%; enhances oxygen utilization and lung function
Mushroom Therapy	Agarikon	20%; expands lung capacity and reduces coughing

Therapy	Solution	Details
Animal Organ Therapy	Lung	29%; strengthens respiratory function and airway health
Amino Acid Therapy	NAC	21%; breaks down mucus and improves lung function

To learn what research and real-world experience reveal about each of these solutions, and which one might be a good fit for you, see the corresponding therapy books in The Medicine-Free, Illness-Free Series.

Environmental and Seasonal Sensitivities

Allergies occur when the immune system overreacts to harmless substances such as pollen, pet dander, dust, or certain foods. This overreaction triggers inflammation, leading to nasal congestion, sneezing, itchy eyes, and respiratory discomfort. For many people, seasonal allergies can significantly impact daily life, while chronic allergies may result in persistent airway irritation, mucus buildup, and sinus inflammation. Although antihistamines are commonly used for symptom relief, natural therapies offer long-term immune balance and symptom reduction without drowsiness or dependency.

Top Solutions for Allergies

Astragalus (9%) – Relieves nasal congestion and reduces allergy-related inflammation by modulating the immune response. Scientific support: Astragalus is a well-known adaptogen with anti-inflammatory and immune-regulating properties that help ease allergy symptoms.

Oregano Oil (9%) – Acts as a natural antihistamine and decongestant, helping clear airways and reduce sinus pressure. Scientific support: Oregano oil contains carvacrol and thymol, compounds shown to reduce histamine response and support respiratory comfort during allergic reactions.

Lung (14%) – Reduces airway inflammation triggered by allergens, promoting clearer breathing and less congestion. Scientific support: Lung glandulars deliver bioavailable peptides that help calm airway inflammation and decrease mucus production linked to allergic reactions.

Thymus (23%) – Modulates immune function to reduce hypersensitivity and excessive inflammation. Scientific support: Thymic peptides help regulate T-cell activity and immune response, reducing overreactions to allergens.

Summary Table: Allergies

Therapy	Solution	Details
Herbal Therapy	Astragalus	9%; relieves nasal congestion and allergic reactions
Herbal Therapy	Oregano Oil	9%; provides antihistamine and decongestant support
Animal Organ Therapy	Lung	14%; reduces airway inflammation linked to allergies
Animal Organ Therapy	Thymus	23%; modulates immune response to reduce hypersensitivity

To learn what research and real-world experience reveal about each of these solutions, and which one might be a good fit for you, see the corresponding therapy books in The Medicine-Free, Illness-Free Series.

Sinus Pressure and Respiratory Irritation

Sinusitis refers to inflammation of the sinus cavities, often caused by infections, chronic allergies, or exposure to environmental irritants. Inflamed sinuses can trap mucus and bacteria, resulting in pressure, nasal congestion, facial pain, and headaches. When left unaddressed, chronic sinusitis may lead to long-term respiratory discomfort and repeated infections. Natural therapies support relief by reducing inflammation, clearing mucus, and enhancing upper respiratory health.

Top Solutions for Sinus Support

Elderberry (17%) – Reduces respiratory infections that often trigger sinus inflammation and congestion. Scientific support: Elderberry is rich in flavonoids with antiviral and anti-inflammatory properties, supporting the immune system and respiratory tract.

Oregano Oil (9%) – Provides powerful antimicrobial and decongestant effects, helping clear nasal passages and relieve sinus pressure. Scientific support: Oregano oil contains carvacrol and thymol, compounds shown to combat sinus-related pathogens and reduce inflammation.

Lung (21%) – Improves respiratory function and promotes better sinus drainage, easing breathing and reducing discomfort. Scientific support: Lung extracts offer peptides and nutrients that enhance immune resilience and support the health of the upper respiratory system.

Summary Table: Sinus Health and Pressure Relief

Therapy	Solution	Details
Herbal Therapy	Elderberry	17%; reduces respiratory infections and sinus issues
Herbal Therapy	Oregano Oil	9%; provides decongestant and antimicrobial support
Animal Organ Therapy	Lung	21%; improves respiratory function and sinus drainage

To learn what research and real-world experience reveal about each of these solutions, and which one might be a good fit for you, see the corresponding therapy books in The Medicine-Free, Illness-Free Series.

Metabolic Health

Metabolic health refers to the body's ability to efficiently regulate blood sugar, insulin levels, fat metabolism, and energy balance. When metabolic processes are disrupted, it can lead to challenges such as weight gain, blood sugar instability, insulin resistance, and fatigue. Over time, poor metabolic function increases the risk of developing conditions such as metabolic syndrome, type 2 diabetes, and cardiovascular issues.

Factors contributing to metabolic dysfunction include high blood glucose, low insulin sensitivity, chronic inflammation, and hormonal imbalances. These imbalances can make it more difficult to maintain a healthy weight, sustain energy levels, and support long-term wellness.

While conventional approaches often rely on medications such as insulin, metformin, or appetite suppressants, natural therapies provide supportive alternatives. These approaches aim to promote metabolic balance by improving insulin sensitivity, enhancing fat metabolism, and supporting the body's energy regulation systems. The following pages explore research-backed natural solutions for promoting optimal metabolic function and restoring internal balance.

Blood Sugar Balance and Insulin Sensitivity

Blood sugar imbalance is a common metabolic concern and may result from insulin resistance, low insulin production, or poor glucose utilization. When left unaddressed, chronically elevated blood sugar can impact energy levels, weight regulation, and long-term health. Supporting healthy blood sugar through nutrition, movement, and targeted supplementation may help promote balanced glucose metabolism and reduce reliance on medications.

Natural therapies work by improving insulin sensitivity, supporting pancreatic function, and enhancing glucose uptake into cells. These approaches may help maintain steady energy, reduce cravings, and protect metabolic health over time.

Top Solutions for Blood Sugar Support

Ceylon Cinnamon (43%) – Improves insulin sensitivity and stabilizes blood sugar levels. Scientific support: Compounds in Ceylon cinnamon enhance insulin function and glucose metabolism, reducing blood glucose levels and supporting type 2 diabetes management.

Maitake (9%) – Enhances insulin function and supports metabolic health. Scientific support: Maitake mushrooms contain beta-glucans that help slow glucose absorption, improve insulin response, and regulate body weight.

Pancreas (12%) – Supports insulin-related functions and helps control blood sugar. Scientific support: Pancreatic extracts provide enzymes and hormone precursors that assist in insulin production and digestive regulation, promoting better glucose control.

Summary Table: Blood Sugar Support

Therapy	Solution	Details
Herbal Therapy	Ceylon Cinnamon	43%; improves insulin sensitivity and stabilizes glucose levels
Mushroom Therapy	Maitake	9%; enhances insulin function and metabolic health

Therapy	Solution	Details
Animal Organ Therapy	Pancreas	12%; supports insulin-related functions and glucose control

To learn what research and real-world experience reveal about each of these solutions, and which one might be a good fit for you, see the corresponding therapy books in The Medicine-Free, Illness-Free Series.

Weight Management and Appetite Control

Effective weight management relies on balanced metabolism, appetite regulation, and efficient fat utilization. Many individuals face challenges such as cravings, low energy, or slow metabolism due to hormonal imbalances, digestive inefficiencies, or insulin resistance. Natural solutions support the body's internal systems by promoting fat metabolism, curbing excessive hunger, and restoring metabolic equilibrium.

Top Solutions for Weight Management

Ceylon Cinnamon (21%) – Helps suppress appetite and reduce cravings by influencing satiety hormones. Scientific support: Ceylon cinnamon improves insulin sensitivity and regulates blood sugar levels, which helps reduce hunger signals and supports better weight control.

Carnitine (22%) – Enhances fat metabolism and supports weight loss by increasing energy production from fat stores. Scientific support: Carnitine transports fatty acids into the mitochondria where they are burned for energy, boosting fat oxidation and aiding in endurance and weight regulation.

Psyllium Husk (10%) – Increases fullness and helps reduce calorie intake. Scientific support: Psyllium absorbs water and expands in the stomach, promoting satiety, slowing gastric emptying, and decreasing overall food consumption.

Maca (7%) – Supports healthy weight gain and improves body composition. Scientific support: Maca has been shown to help increase lean muscle mass and support hormone balance, which may aid in improving weight in individuals with low body weight or poor muscle tone.

Summary Table: Weight Management

Therapy	Solution	Details
Herbal Therapy	Ceylon Cinnamon	21%; helps suppress appetite and reduce cravings
Amino Acid Therapy	Carnitine	22%; enhances fat metabolism for weight control
HOPED Protocol	Psyllium Husk	10%; increases fullness and reduces calorie intake
Herbal Therapy	Maca	7%; supports healthy weight gain and body composition

To learn what research and real-world experience reveal about each of these solutions, and which one might be a good fit for you, see the corresponding therapy books in The Medicine-Free, Illness-Free Series.

Metabolic Resilience

Metabolic syndrome is a cluster of conditions that significantly raise the risk of diabetes, cardiovascular disease, and stroke. It is typically defined by a combination of high blood sugar, elevated blood pressure, excess abdominal fat, and abnormal cholesterol levels. A sluggish metabolism often contributes to these imbalances, leading to weight gain, insulin resistance, and inconsistent energy levels. Supporting metabolic function, particularly through thyroid health, plays a key role in restoring energy, regulating weight, and improving overall resilience.

Top Solutions for Metabolic Syndrome

Thyroid (15%) – Enhances metabolic rate and energy production by supporting thyroid hormone activity. Scientific support: The thyroid gland regulates metabolism, body temperature, and energy balance, making thyroid supplementation beneficial for individuals with metabolic syndrome and sluggish metabolic function.

Summary Table: Metabolic Syndrome

Therapy	Solution	Details
Animal Organ Therapy	Thyroid	15%; enhances metabolic rate and energy production

To learn what research and real-world experience reveal about this solution, and whether it might be a good fit for you, see the corresponding therapy books in The Medicine-Free, Illness-Free Series.

Hormonal Health and Endocrine Balance

Hormonal balance plays a central role in metabolism, reproductive function, emotional well-being, and overall vitality. When hormones become disrupted due to aging, stress, dietary factors, or other imbalances, individuals may experience symptoms such as fatigue, weight changes, mood fluctuations, irregular menstrual cycles, fertility challenges, or slowed metabolism.

Three of the most commonly experienced hormonal challenges include thyroid-related issues, menopause transitions, and symptoms associated with polycystic ovary syndrome (PCOS).

While conventional treatments such as hormone replacement therapy (HRT), thyroid medications, and oral contraceptives are frequently used, these options may carry side effects and often do not address underlying nutritional or functional imbalances. Natural therapies offer a more integrative approach by providing key hormonal building blocks, essential cofactors, and adaptogenic support to help gently restore endocrine balance and support long-term wellness.

Hormonal Transitions and Menopausal Support

Menopause is a natural phase of life that may bring changes in mood, energy, sleep, and physical comfort as estrogen and progesterone levels shift. These hormonal fluctuations can influence a woman's sense of balance and overall vitality. Rather than masking these changes, some individuals explore natural options that help the body adapt to this transition with greater ease and resilience.

Top Solutions for Menopausal Support

Female Organs (9%) – Commonly used to support the body's natural rhythms during perimenopause. Scientific support: Female glandular extracts contain nutrient cofactors and hormone precursors that may assist in maintaining balance through hormonal transitions.

Female Organs (15%) – May help promote emotional steadiness and reduce sensitivity to daily stressors during midlife. Scientific support: These extracts offer components believed to support estrogen and progesterone balance in non-clinical settings.

Female Organs (8%) – Selected by some users to support energy and vitality during life stage transitions. Scientific support: Female organ supplements are rich in nutrients that may contribute to overall endocrine system nourishment.

Summary Table: Menopause Transition Support

Therapy	Solution	Details
Animal Organ Therapy	Female Organs	9%; helps regulate menstrual cycles and reduce irregularities
Animal Organ Therapy	Female Organs	15%; reduces mood swings and promotes emotional balance
Animal Organ Therapy	Female Organs	8%; improves endocrine function and hormone balance

Note: When a single solution appears in multiple lines, like Animal Female Organ supplement (Uterus and Ovaries), each entry reflects a different user-reported benefit or pattern of use. This format helps illustrate the range of experiences and outcomes observed. For more details on how each solution works and how to use it effectively, see the corresponding therapy book in *The Medicine-Free, Illness-Free Series.*

To learn what research and real-world experience reveal about this solution, and whether it might be a good fit for you, see the corresponding therapy books in The Medicine-Free, Illness-Free Series.

Reproductive Endocrine Imbalance

Hormonal fluctuations can affect a woman's reproductive rhythm, energy, mood, and metabolic function. Irregular menstrual cycles, occasional ovarian discomfort, and hormone-related symptoms such as bloating or skin imbalance are increasingly common concerns. These shifts may be influenced by stress, nutritional gaps, metabolic changes, or lifestyle habits.

Natural therapies can help support reproductive balance by promoting healthy hormone signaling, encouraging regular menstrual patterns, and fostering ovarian and uterine wellness. These approaches have been traditionally used to support female health through various life stages and are now gaining interest for their broader role in endocrine support.

Top Solutions for Reproductive Cycle Support

Maca (37%) – Supports hormone balance and promotes menstrual regularity. Scientific support: Maca is traditionally used to nourish the hypothalamic-pituitary axis and support estrogen-progesterone rhythm, helping promote hormonal harmony and energy.

Female Organs (8%) – Selected by some users to support reproductive cycle and hormonal balance. Scientific support: Female organ supplements are rich in nutrients that may contribute to overall endocrine system nourishment.

Summary Table: Reproductive Cycle Support

Therapy	Solution	Details
Herbal Therapy	Maca	37%; balances hormones and regulates menstrual cycles
Animal Organ Therapy	Female Organs	8%; improves endocrine function and hormone balance

To learn what research and real-world experience reveal about each of these solutions, and which one might be a good fit for you, see the corresponding therapy books in The Medicine-Free, Illness-Free Series.

Thyroid Support and Energy Regulation

The thyroid gland plays a central role in regulating energy, metabolism, and hormonal rhythms throughout the body. When thyroid activity is not optimal, individuals may experience changes in energy levels, weight, mood, and skin appearance. These imbalances may be influenced by stress, nutrient status, environmental exposures, or aging.

Natural therapies may help support thyroid health by nourishing glandular function and providing key nutrients involved in hormone synthesis. This approach is designed to encourage metabolic balance and promote steady, sustained energy.

Top Solutions for Thyroid Support

Thyroid (46%) – Supports thyroid health, energy regulation, and hormonal balance. Scientific support: Thyroid supplements derived from glandular tissue provide bioavailable thyroid nutrients along with cofactors such as iodine and selenium, which are essential for supporting the body's natural thyroid hormone production and overall metabolic vitality.

Summary Table: Thyroid Support

Therapy	Solution	Details
Animal Organ Therapy	Thyroid	46%; supports thyroid function, metabolic health, and hormone balance

To learn what research and real-world experience reveal about this solution, and whether it might be a good fit for you, see the corresponding therapy books in The Medicine-Free, Illness-Free Series.

Bone and Joint Health

Bone and joint health are vital for maintaining strength, stability, and freedom of movement. Over time, natural changes in the body, such as reduced bone mineral density and cartilage wear, may contribute to decreased flexibility, stiffness, and increased vulnerability to discomfort or mobility limitations. Lifestyle factors including poor nutrition, hormonal fluctuations, and low physical activity levels may further affect musculoskeletal resilience.

Structural changes in bones and joints can be influenced by nutrient imbalances, hormonal shifts, or age-related changes that impact bone density and joint function. Many individuals seek additional support for maintaining bone integrity and joint mobility as part of their long-term wellness goals.

While conventional approaches often include calcium supplementation, physical therapy, or medications, natural therapies offer additional options. These approaches focus on providing structural nutrients, collagen-building support, and co-factors that may help nourish bones and promote joint comfort.

Let me know when you're ready for the table or the condition-specific rewrites (e.g., *Osteoporosis*, *Joint Mobility*, etc.) that follow this section.

Bone Strength and Density

Many individuals seek support for maintaining strong, resilient bones as they age, especially when concerns arise about declining bone density or structural integrity. Healthy bone formation depends on the body's ability to absorb and utilize essential minerals like calcium, phosphorus, and magnesium, along with collagen-building nutrients. Natural therapies can support the body's natural processes for bone remodeling, mineralization, and skeletal strength.

Top Solutions for Bone Density and Structural Support

Bone and Marrow (12%) – Supports bone density and skeletal resilience. Scientific support: Bone and marrow supplements provide essential minerals like calcium, phosphorus, and magnesium, along with collagen precursors that support structural bone integrity and help maintain flexibility and resilience.

Vitamin D (20%) – Enhances calcium absorption and promotes bone health. Scientific support: Vitamin D is crucial for the body's ability to absorb calcium and support proper bone mineralization. Research shows that maintaining adequate Vitamin D levels supports skeletal strength and mineral balance.

Summary Table: Bone Density and Strength Support

Therapy	Solution	Details
Animal Organ Therapy	Bone and Marrow	12%; supports bone density and structural resilience
HOPED Protocol	Vitamin D	20%; enhances calcium absorption and promotes healthy bone metabolism

To learn what research and real-world experience reveal about each of these solutions, and which one might be a good fit for you, see the corresponding therapy books in The Medicine-Free, Illness-Free Series.

Joint Integrity and Mobility

Joints play a vital role in flexibility, mobility, and cushioning, allowing the body to move comfortably and efficiently. Over time, natural wear and tear can affect cartilage and connective tissues, leading to stiffness and reduced range of motion. Supporting joint lubrication, collagen structure, and connective tissue integrity helps promote long-term joint comfort and mobility.

Top Solutions for Joint Strength and Cartilage Support

Cartilage (61%) – Supports joint mobility and comfort. Scientific support: Beef cartilage is rich in type II collagen and glycosaminoglycans (GAGs), which have been shown to support cartilage health, enhance joint lubrication, and promote normal joint function.

Collagen (25%) – Helps reduce stiffness and support joint elasticity. Scientific support: Type II collagen contributes to joint cushioning and structural support, aiding comfort during physical activity and daily movement.

Cartilage (16%) – Eases occasional knee stiffness and supports joint flexibility. Scientific support: Type II collagen and chondroitin sulfate in beef cartilage help maintain joint tissue and encourage healthy mobility.

Bone and Marrow (17%) – Promotes smoother joint movement and flexibility. Scientific support: Bone marrow contains collagen and GAGs that support connective tissue health and joint lubrication.

Cartilage (16%) – Supports long-term cartilage integrity. Scientific support: Undenatured type II collagen and other compounds in cartilage help maintain healthy cartilage through the body's natural repair processes.

Bone and Marrow (10%) – Aids flexibility and joint comfort. Scientific support: Nutrients and structural proteins found in bone marrow help nourish connective tissues and support cartilage resilience.

Summary Table: Joint Strength and Flexibility

Therapy	Solution	Details
Animal Organ	Cartilage	61%; supports joint mobility and comfort
Animal Organ	Collagen	25%; helps reduce joint stiffness and promote elasticity
Animal Organ	Cartilage	16%; eases occasional knee stiffness and supports flexibility
Animal Organ	Bone and Marrow	17%; promotes joint flexibility and movement comfort
Animal Organ	Cartilage	16%; helps maintain long-term cartilage integrity
Animal Organ	Bone and Marrow	10%; supports cartilage resilience and joint comfort

Note: When a single solution appears in multiple lines, such as cartilage, each entry reflects a different user-reported benefit or pattern of use. This format helps illustrate the range of experiences and outcomes observed. For more details on how each solution works and how to use it effectively, see the corresponding therapy book in *The Medicine-Free, Illness-Free Series*.

To learn what research and real-world experience reveal about each of these solutions, and which one might be a good fit for you, see the corresponding therapy books in The Medicine-Free, Illness-Free Series.

Integrative Daily Wellness Routine

Throughout this book, we've explored a wide range of natural therapies designed to support specific health goals, from digestive challenges and immune system support to hormonal imbalances and energy concerns. While these targeted approaches can be helpful when specific needs arise, long-term vitality is often supported by consistent, everyday habits that work with the body's natural rhythms. Instead of reacting to discomfort after it appears, a proactive daily routine may help the body function more efficiently and maintain wellness over time.

This is where a daily wellness routine becomes valuable, not just to address occasional symptoms, but to promote balance, strengthen resilience, and help the body perform at its best. In *The Medicine-Free, Illness-Free Series*, we've introduced several categories of natural health support: herbal therapy, mushroom therapy, organ therapy, amino acid therapy, detoxification therapy, grounding practices, and the HOPED Protocol, which includes High Fiber, Omega-3s and Antioxidants, Probiotics, Enzymes, and Vitamin D. These tools can each offer meaningful support on their own, but when integrated thoughtfully into daily life, their benefits may be amplified through synergy and consistency.

Each therapy plays a distinct role. Mushroom therapy is often used to support immune resilience, brain function, and the body's natural defenses. Organ therapy may offer bioavailable nutrients to support organ function, hormonal balance, and digestive health. Amino acid therapy supports muscle repair, neurotransmitter production, mood stability, and energy metabolism. Grounding therapy, including the use of grounding mats or sheets, may help support physical relaxation, healthy inflammation response, and improved sleep patterns. Herbal therapy offers support for a wide range of everyday wellness goals, from energy and focus to digestion, mood, and aging. The HOPED protocol provides core nutrients that many people find essential for gut health, metabolic balance, and long-term immune function.

By bringing these therapies together in a practical, well-structured daily routine, you can create a system that supports your body naturally and consistently, one that helps maintain balance, reduce stress, and promote healthy function across all systems. For instance, grounding tools can be used effortlessly while you sleep, supporting rest and recovery overnight. Mushroom and organ-based supplements can be taken alongside meals to simplify implementation. Amino acids may be helpful before or after physical activity to support muscle recovery and stamina. Adaptogenic herbs such as Ashwagandha or calming mushrooms like Reishi can be used in the evening to support emotional balance and sleep quality.

The goal of this approach is not to overwhelm, but to create a simple structure you can personalize over time. You may begin with just a few key additions, such as a grounding mat at night or adding a mushroom blend to your morning routine, and build from there. What matters most is consistency and a willingness to listen to your body and make adjustments based on how you feel.

The best way to experience the benefits of these natural therapies is to integrate them gradually and consistently. While health goals vary from person to person, many people find that having a reliable daily rhythm helps reinforce progress, maintain energy throughout the day, and support overall well-being. In this chapter, you'll find a clear and flexible daily routine designed to help you begin. Whether your goal is to increase energy, support immune health, improve digestion, balance mood, or simply feel more grounded and refreshed, this template offers a practical foundation you can adapt to your unique lifestyle.

To help you seamlessly incorporate these therapies into your everyday life, we've designed a clear and easy-to-follow daily routine example. This routine focuses on enhancing energy, focus, and immune health in the morning and afternoon, supporting strength and recovery in the later part of the day, and promoting rest and sleep quality in the evening. You can use this template to begin building your own customized wellness rhythm, one that supports your goals both now and into the future.

Morning / Breakfast: Start Your Day with Energy and Focus

Your morning routine sets the tone for the entire day. By incorporating specific therapies and supplements, you can boost your energy levels, enhance cognitive function, and strengthen your immune system right from the start.

Therapy	Solution	Direction	Benefits
Herbal	Rhodiola Rosea	Take as supplement with breakfast.	Enhances energy levels, improves focus and cognitive functions.
Mushroom	Turkey Tail	Take as supplements with breakfast.	Boosts immune function, enhances cognitive performance, and increases physical energy.
Animal Organ	Beef Liver	Take as supplements with breakfast.	Provides dense nutrition to nourish internal organs, balance hormones, and supply essential digestive enzymes.

Therapy	Solution	Direction	Benefits
HOPED	Vitamin D, Shilajit	Take as supplements with breakfast.	Provides vitamin and minerals, supports bone health, immune function, and enhances overall energy levels.

Although this is a comprehensive list of recommended supplements for the morning, you may decide to take only a subset of it. E.g. only focus on Mushroom supplements and/or Beef Organ supplements.

Noon/ Lunch Maintain Focus and Strengthen Immunity

Your lunch routine should sustain the energy and focus you've built up in the morning while continuing to support your immune system. Incorporate antioxidants and maintain your organ health with additional supplements.

Therapy	Solution	Direction	Benefits
Herbal	Turmeric	Take as supplement with lunch.	Reduce inflammation and discomfort
Mushroom	Turkey Tail	Take as supplements with lunch.	Continues to support immune health and cognitive performance.
Animal Organ	Beef Pancreas	Take as supplements with lunch.	Maintains nutrient levels and supports digestion and ongoing organ health.
HOPED	Omega-3 Fish Oil	Take as supplements with lunch.	Protects cells from oxidative stress, supports heart and brain health, anti-aging, and enhances immune function.

Afternoon: Enhance Muscle Growth and Endurance

In the afternoon, focus on supporting your muscles and maintaining your energy levels, especially if you engage in physical activity such as exercises. Essential amino acids not only play a crucial role in muscle synthesis and recovery but also enhance the health of neurotransmitters and mood.

Therapy	Solution	Direction	Benefits
Amino Acid	Essential Amino Acids (EAA)	Consume EAA supplements before or after your workout, or at afternoon break	Supports protein synthesis, muscle growth, strength, endurance, and overall physical performance.

Evening/ Dinner: Promote Relaxation and Prepare for Restful Sleep

Your evening routine should help you wind down, reduce inflammation, and prepare your body for a restful night. Incorporate relaxing herbs and antioxidants to support overall well-being.

Therapy	Solution	Direction	Benefits
Mushroom Therapy	Reishi	Take as supplements with dinner.	Promotes restful sleep, reduces stress, and supports immune health.
Animal Organ	Beef Pancreas	Take as supplements with dinner.	Provides essential digestive enzymes, blood sugar regulation, and supports overnight organ health.
HOPED	Fiber	Take as supplements with dinner.	Maintains gut health and promotes regular bowel movements.

Bedtime: Settle Your Digestive Track and Enhance Sleep Quality

Before bed, focus on maintaining gut health and ensuring a restful night's sleep. Incorporate probiotics and fiber to support digestion and cleansing and use grounding therapy to enhance sleep quality.

Therapy	Solution	Direction	Benefits
HOPED	Probiotics	Take probiotic supplements and fiber supplements before bed.	Maintains gut health, supports digestion, and promotes regular bowel movements overnight.
Grounding	Grounding Mat	Use a grounding mat or sheet while you sleep.	Continuously reduces inflammation, promotes healing, and enhances sleep quality.

Customizing Your Daily Routine

While this example routine provides a structured framework for integrating various therapies, it's essential to personalize it based on your specific health goals, lifestyle, and individual needs. Here's how you can tailor this routine to create a personalized health regimen:

Assess Your Health Goals: Determine whether your primary focus is on boosting energy, enhancing cognitive function, strengthening the immune system, supporting muscle growth, or promoting relaxation and better sleep. Whether you are to support existing health concerns or to maintain long term health.

Reference Specific Area of concerns: For targeted health concerns, refer to previous chapters to identify which therapies and supplements may help.

Select a Subset of Therapies

Not every therapy or supplement may fit into your daily routine. Choose only the ones that align with your goals and are feasible for your lifestyle. For example, if you're focused on stress reduction, prioritize grounding techniques and Reishi mushrooms. If immunity is your goal, focus on mushroom supplements like Turkey Tail, and Vitamin D.

Adjust Dosages and Timing: Based on your individual health status and professional advice, modify the dosages and timing of each therapy to optimize their effectiveness.

Monitor and Adapt: Pay attention to how your body responds to the integrated routine. Make adjustments as necessary and consult healthcare professionals to ensure the regimen remains safe and effective.

Building Daily Routine Gradually

The daily supplement routine outlined above is designed to provide a strong foundation for overall health maintenance, supporting key areas such as immune resilience, cognitive function, emotional well-being, and physical vitality. While the routine is comprehensive and highly beneficial, it's important to recognize that everyone's body is unique. Jumping into a fully loaded routine all at once can feel overwhelming, both physically and mentally. Instead, we recommend a gradual approach to building your personalized regimen and below is an example.

Why a Gradual Approach Works Best

Introducing new supplements into your routine one at a time allows your body to adjust and respond. It gives you the opportunity to observe how each supplement affects your energy levels, focus, mood, sleep, or any specific health goals. This step-by-step process also minimizes the risk of potential side effects and ensures you're only including supplements that provide noticeable benefits for you.

Moreover, taking this approach over the span of several weeks allows you to fine-tune the routine to meet your individual needs, making it more sustainable in the long term.

How to Gradually Adopt the Daily Routine

Building a comprehensive daily supplement routine is a powerful way to support your overall health and well-being, but it's important to do so in a way that makes it sustainable and allows you to understand how each element affects your body. A step-by-step approach, focusing on one therapy at a time, is the best way to adopt the routine gradually and effectively.

Start with One Therapy at a Time

The following order provides a structured path to gradually build your routine. This allows you to introduce each therapy individually, observe its effects, and determine how well it supports your health:

Begin with Mushroom Therapy

Mushrooms are some of the most versatile and potent supplements for immune health, cognitive support, and energy levels. Start by adding Lion's Mane for cognitive enhancement, followed by Turkey Tail for immune support and cancer prevention, and then Cordyceps for energy and stamina. Take one at a time for couple days days before introducing the next. Finally, add Reishi in the evening for relaxation and stress reduction.

Incorporate Animal Organ Therapy

Once you've experienced the benefits of mushrooms, start adding organ supplements. Begin with Liver or Organ Complex, as they provide essential nutrients for overall vitality. Gradually include specific organs like Heart, Kidney, or Pancreas based on your individual needs. For example, Kidney can be helpful for histamine intolerance, while Pancreas supports digestive health and blood sugar regulation.

Add Herbal Therapies

After stabilizing your mushroom and organ therapies, begin introducing herbal supplements. Start with Rhodiola Rosea in the morning to improve focus and energy. Gradually add Turmeric for its anti-inflammatory and pain-killer properties and Ashwagandha in the evening to promote relaxation and balance stress levels. Introduce one herb at a time to evaluate its effects.

Incorporate Essential Amino Acids (EAA)

You may add **EAA** to your routine any time during the process, to support neurotransmitter synthesis, muscle recovery, and overall energy. These are especially beneficial if you exercise regularly. Begin by taking EAAs in the afternoon, or any time before or after your workout, and monitor how they enhance your physical and mental performance.

Try Grounding Therapy

Once your supplements are stabilized, consider adding Grounding Therapy by using a grounding mat during sleep. This practice helps reduce inflammation, improve sleep quality, and promote overall relaxation. Since grounding requires no additional effort, it's a simple yet impactful addition to your daily routine.

Vitamin D and Omega-3

These two key supplements can be added at any time during your journey. Vitamin D supports immunity, mood, and bone health, while Omega-3 strengthens neuronal membranes and reduces inflammation. Both are essential foundational elements and integrate seamlessly with any phase of the routine.

Summary of the Integrative Daily Routine

The table below summarizes the foundational daily routine example for your reference.

Therapy	Breakfast	Lunch	Afternoon	Dinner	Bed Time
Herbal	Rhodiola Rosea	Turmeric			
Mushroom	Turkey Tail	Turkey Tail		Reishi	
Animal Organ	Beef Liver	Beef Pancreas		Beef Pancreas	
Amino Acid			EAA		
HOPED	Vitamin D, Shilajit	Fish Oil		Fiber	Probiotics
Grounding					Grounding Mat

This example routine is intended to illustrate how various natural solutions can be combined to support overall wellness. Your ideal daily plan may differ based on your personal goals, sensitivities, and lifestyle factors. To determine which solutions may best fit your unique needs, be sure to explore the detailed information provided in each corresponding therapy book in *The Medicine-Free, Illness-Free Series.* Each book offers in-depth guidance on how the solution works, what real users are saying, and how to use it effectively. By learning about the science-informed mechanisms, user-reported benefits, and practical usage patterns, you'll be better equipped to create a personalized wellness routine that supports your long-term vitality and balance.

A Final Word: The Journey to Vibrant Health

As we come to the conclusion of *Integrative Therapies for Everyday Health*, one message stands out: effective, approachable solutions for everyday wellness are within your reach. This book has introduced you to a wide range of evidence-informed strategies, grounded in both scientific research and real-world experience, that address common concerns like fatigue, stress, poor digestion, hormonal fluctuations, and immune imbalance.

Rather than relying on extreme interventions or one-size-fits-all prescriptions, this guide has offered a flexible reference for working with the body's natural systems. You've explored how integrative approaches, including herbal remedies, medicinal mushrooms, organ-based nutrition, amino acids, grounding practices, targeted detox protocols, and the HOPED framework, can work together to nourish resilience, restore balance, and elevate daily function.

To help you apply what you've learned, we've included a single, comprehensive daily routine example that you can reference and customize to fit your needs. This routine demonstrates how small, consistent steps, when integrated into your daily habits, can contribute to sustained energy, resilience, and long-term wellness.

This book is part of *The Medicine-Free, Illness-Free Series*, which includes companion volumes focused on individual therapy areas: Diet & Lifestyle, Herbal Therapy, Mushroom Therapy, Animal Organ Therapy, Amino Acid Therapy, the HOPED Protocol, Detoxification, and Grounding Therapy. Each one expands on the solutions you've seen here, providing deeper guidance on what the science shows, what real people experience, and how to make it work in your life.

No matter where you are in your journey, know that vibrant health is not out of reach. By choosing to support your body naturally, through nourishment, rhythm, and restoration, you are honoring its built-in intelligence and regenerative power. Each supplement you take, grounding habit you practice, or plant-based therapy you explore is a step toward greater wellness that accumulates over time.

Thank you for allowing this book to be part of your journey. May it continue to serve as a practical, empowering resource, helping you respond to everyday health concerns with clarity, confidence, and care.

To explore more solutions or receive personalized guidance, visit AshiHealing.com.

About the Author

Dr. Forest Yin (Jie Yin) is a licensed acupuncturist, herbalist, and Doctor of Acupuncture and Oriental Medicine (DAOM). He serves as a professor and doctoral advisor at the University of East West Medicine (UEWM) and is the founder of Ashi Healing and Acupuncture Inc. With extensive experience in Traditional Chinese Medicine (TCM) and natural health, Dr. Yin integrates a wide range of holistic therapies, forming the foundation of *The Medicine-Free, Illness-Free Series.*

Before devoting his career fully to natural healing, Dr. Yin worked in the high-tech and financial sectors with both large corporations and fast-paced startups. These experiences gave him firsthand insight into the chronic stress and burnout common in modern life. Inspired to seek sustainable strategies for long-term wellness, he turned to the wisdom of nature and the depth of Chinese medicine.

Dr. Yin's clinical experience and ongoing research have helped shape practical wellness protocols that focus on balance, energy, and lifestyle-based health support. His work emphasizes simple, science-informed approaches that align with the body's natural rhythms and support overall resilience.

Driven by a mission to empower others, he created *The Medicine-Free, Illness-Free Series* to share accessible natural strategies that fit seamlessly into busy lives. His approach blends ancient healing principles with modern insight, helping people feel more energized, focused, and in tune with their long-term health goals.

Continue Your Healing Journey

This book is just the beginning. True wellness is a lifelong journey, and you don't have to walk it alone. The Ashi Healing ecosystem is here to support you every step of the way with personalized guidance, nature-based solutions, and a shared mission: to help more people experience the benefits of natural health.

Personalized Virtual Consultation

If you're ready for expert guidance tailored to your specific needs, you can schedule a private virtual consultation with Dr. Forest Yin at AshiHealing.com. These one-on-one sessions offer a personalized supplement and herbal plan based on your current wellness goals, lifestyle, and health history, helping you create a sustainable path forward using time-tested, natural approaches.

In-Person Consultation and Acupuncture

If you're located in the San Francisco Bay Area, Dr. Yin also provides in-person consultations and acupuncture sessions at the University of East West Medicine (UEWM) campus in Sunnyvale, California, where he also teaches in the doctoral program for Traditional Chinese Medicine. This serene, professional setting offers a welcoming space for personalized care. All visits, virtual or in-person, can be scheduled through AshiHealing.com.

Supplement Recommendation Plans

Each wellness protocol discussed in this book has a corresponding supplement plan available on Fullscript, featuring practitioner-trusted, food-based formulas. These curated plans make it easy to take action without guesswork, offering clear, guided steps for nutritional support.

You can access them directly at:

https://us.fullscript.com/welcome/ashi-healing,

or simply start from AshiHealing.com.

Explore the Complete Book Series

This book is part of *The Medicine-Free, Illness-Free Series*, a 10-book collection designed to help you support your long-term health and vitality through natural methods. Each volume introduces a unique modality—from herbs and mushrooms to detoxification, grounding, amino acids, and more—so you can build your wellness path one step at a time.

Refer to the Series Overview chapter or visit AshiHealing.com to explore the full collection.

Support the Natural Health Movement

If this book has inspired you, and you believe more people should have access to clear, trustworthy information about natural health, consider supporting our mission.

The Ashi Healing Foundation *(AshiHealing.org)* is a nonprofit organization dedicated to public education, natural health awareness, and holistic wellness outreach. Your tax-deductible donation helps expand access to these tools and empowers more individuals to explore safe, evidence-informed approaches to well-being.

To contribute, visit AshiHealing.org and join the movement for a healthier, freer world.

Connect and Stay Inspired

Your healing journey doesn't end here.

Follow **Dr. Forest Yin** for more healing stories, tips, and inspiration:

Instagram, TikTok, YouTube, and X: @DrForestYin

Facebook: @DrForestYin1

LinkedIn: linkedin.com/in/forest-yin

Ready to Take the Next Step?

Scan the QR code below to visit AshiHealing.com, your starting point for virtual consultations, supplement plans, and more resources.

Your journey toward sustainable, natural wellness begins now.

Made in the USA
Monee, IL
08 November 2026

68007848R00100